PRAISE FOR REGENERATE YOUR BRAIN

"While we live in a time of ever increasing rates of brain related diseases, from Alzheimer's to depression to attention deficit disorder, it's surprising to many to learn that to a significant degree, each of us is the arbiter of our brain's destiny. Our day-to-day choices related to the food we eat and the activities in which we engage are powerfully influential in terms of the brain's functionality and resistance to degeneration. And Regenerate Your Brain *eloquently presents not just why these choices matter, but how they can be easily implemented for your better brain. Take control of your brain's destiny - here's how."*

—**David Perlmutter, MD**,
#1 *New York Times* bestselling author of
Grain Brain and *Brain Wash*

"Although the field of neuroscience has made tremendous progress over the past couple of decades, understanding the essential principles of brain function, and putting that knowledge to personal use, is still far more unknown than known. Dr. Jacqueline Chan's new book is the most comprehensive and user-friendly book on this all important subject I have ever come across and I highly recommend it to anyone seeking greater health and happiness."

—**Dr. Jeff Rockwell**, DC, MA, DOMP

"Through her personal journey and evidence-based wellness strategies, Dr. Chan enlightens us with a comprehensive array of practical information and valuable resources. Her holistic approach offers us the ability to heal our bodies and keep our brains active and healthy well into our 70s, 80s and beyond."

—Beth Greer,
Environmental Health Educator and
author of *Super Natural Home*

"Weaving together rigorous science with decades of clinical wisdom, Dr. Jaqueline Chan has written an exquisite book offering a roadmap to a more peaceful mind."

—Shauna Shapiro, PhD,
author of *Good Morning I Love You*

"In Regenerate Your Brain, *Dr. Chan proves that you don't need to live with depression, anger or other negative emotions. She offers a comprehensive, easy-to-use guide that can help you to experience ongoing states of tranquility, happiness and focus. This is a definitive road map to enhance your brain health and overall well-being."*

—Marci Shimoff,
#1 *New York Times* best-selling author of
Chicken Soup for the Woman's Soul and *Happy for No Reason*

"Regenerate Your Brain *provides deep and well researched information along with practical steps for achieving greater brain health, neuroplasticity, longevity and holistic regenerative wellness. I feel smarter already having just read the book and feel improvement in my clarity and overall health from following Dr. Chan's suggestions!*

—Mark Stephen Chasan, CEO,
AWE Global, Inc.

"I opened it up just to take a glance, before I began my very busy day...and could not stop scrolling through and reading more. An hour went by. It is totally fabulous. The book is EXCELLENT and it deserves to be ushered thoughtfully and successfully into the world, where it can help as many people as possible."

—Miranda Macpherson,
spiritual teacher, modern mystic and author

"In this excellent new book on brain health, Dr. Chan offers practical and clear guidance on understanding the mystery of the brain and what you can do to support optimize its functioning. Through her clear guidance based on years of clinical practice, you will find her words illuminate the path to true brain health and genuine well-being and happiness."

—Mark Coleman,
author of *From Suffering to Peace*
and *Make Peace with Your Mind*

REGENERATE
YOUR **BRAIN**

REGENERATE YOUR BRAIN

A Breakthrough Plan To
Restore Your Brilliant Mind

Dr. Jacqueline Chan, DO, MIM

The contents of this book are for informational purposes only. The content is not intended to be a substitute for professional medical advice, diagnosis, or treatment. Always seek the advice of your physician or other qualified health provider with any questions you may have regarding a medical condition.

Jacqueline Susanna Chan, DO
PO Box 35 Miller Avenue 202
Mill Valley, CA 94941

ISBN 978-1-7350387-0-4 (p)
ISBN 978-1-7350387-1-1 (e)

Library of Congress Number: 1735038709 paperback
Library of Congress Number:1735038717 ebook

Edited by Nina Shoroplova—NinaShoroplova.ca
Cover art by Hera Lee
Book interior and ebook design by Amit Dey—amitdey2528@gmail.com
Publishing consulting by Geoff Affleck—geoffaffleck.com

HEA032000 HEALTH & FITNESS / Alternative Therapies
HEA010000 HEALTH & FITNESS / Healthy Living
HEA047000 HEALTH & FITNESS / Body Cleansing & Detoxification
HEA039110 HEALTH & FITNESS / Diseases / Nervous System
OCC010000 BODY, MIND & SPIRIT / Mindfulness & Meditation

DEDICATION

I dedicate this book to my father and grandfather for their marriage to medicine as a noble path of service and to my patients; past, present and future for inspiring me, challenging me and without whom this book would not have had a causative force. Finally, to my brain and central nervous system may you know that all the difficulties you underwent can now give their gifts of wisdom down the path of healing to others so that we can mend together.

CONTENTS

PREFACE

Amidst the eruption of books on neuroscience in recent years, very few are written to cover comprehensive yet foundational health care musts for brain health. These other books may inform you about our concept of "the mind" or explore who we are as conscious beings. They may guide you into a new way to meditate, or expose you to intriguing case studies, therapies, and research discoveries. People are now offering special diets that promote brain health with powerful brain-enhancing supplements or sound-healing strategies. While I was writing this book, people would ask me what it was about. When I replied, "Taking care of our brains," they would often ask me if I was writing about mushroom journeys, the latest nootropic pill they could swallow to make them brilliant, or some form of artificial intelligence they could put on their head to shift brain waves. Not that I'm opposed to any of those, but the truth is so few people are doing even the basic, foundational health care steps for their brains.

When it comes to the brain, there's no single answer. Think about it—our brain has a very complex job. It thinks for us, moves our bodies, and is in charge of all our physiological processes, such as the pace of our heartbeat and our breathing, the release of our hormones, the play of our emotions and memories. It is also the basis of our creative arts and ingenuity. The brain, thus, deserves an equally comprehensive healing approach.

As a holistic physician, one of my gifts is the ability to synergize a wide cross-section of academic disciplines. I realized in writing this book that healing the brain really means we can't leave anything out. I view it as applying a wheel of wellness, with the brain in the center, benefiting from everything else we do in the circumference. If we look at this wheel, we will find it is regenerative, it includes all aspects of good health, and it allows the brain to evolve based on the latest principles of neuroplasticity. This wheel has the following eight sections:

1. Nourishing the brain
2. Balancing healthy hormones
3. Healing leaky gut and leaky brain
4. Cooling brain inflammation
5. Detoxifying for clear cognition
6. Boosting mitochondria and regenerating new neural tissue
7. Soothing the mind
8. Building new neural pathways

Few books dealing with neuroscience or the brain are written with this comprehensive array of wellness strategies. After working with hundreds of patients over the course of twenty-five years, I'm convinced that the ultimate path to harnessing the maximum capacity for our brain's remodeling needs to be an inclusive, whole approach. The spectacular side effect of this approach is that what's good for the brain is good for your entire body. As you heal your body using the wheel of wellness, your ability to navigate complexities in the straightforward way I have laid out provides whole health. It helps your ability to lower your stress response and enhances your ability to have intimate connected relationships, feel more joy, create greater efficiency in your work, clarify your purpose, focus yourself intellectually, create innovative experiences, rest deeply, become emotionally resilient, and in the end, live a deeply fulfilled life.

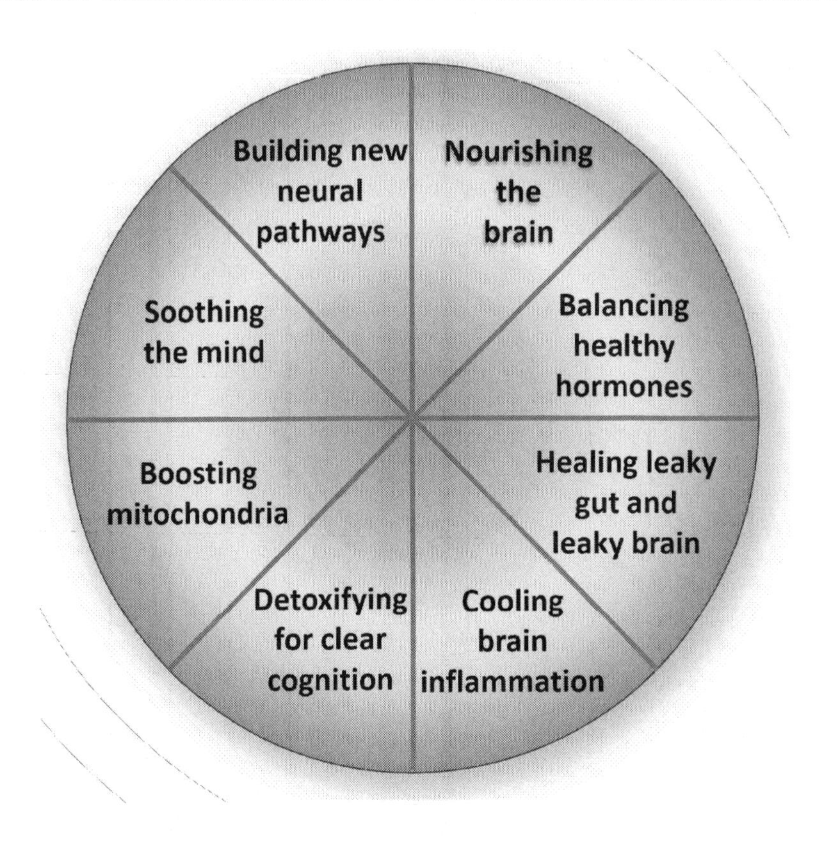

As a physician, I want to help my patients immediately. This is the spirit from which I wrote this book. I thought, *What if all it took was a few hours of reading for people to create an evidence-based, practical, and effective plan for their optimal brain health?* I hope this book explains not only the "why" behind supplement prescriptions and lab work but also the "what and how" with relative ease. I placed some of the research studies in sidebars so that if you want to read this book more quickly, you can skip the research sections for now and come back to them later. I also placed supplement lists, dosages, and a list of labs at the end of each chapter so that you can organize your to-do list in terms of maximizing the tools that help you attain optimal brain health. At the end of the book, I have a resources section that contains links to videos to watch, retreat centers to attend, recipes to cook, and people to contact for certain equipment or supplements I've referenced. The main chapters of the book are geared toward more lengthy physiological explanations behind the "whys and hows" of regenerative brain care.

I have been practicing as a board-certified family physician and board-certified holistic medicine practitioner since 1994. The importance of my education really hit home when I was challenged by several insults to my own brain. In the first chapter of this book, "My Story," I share with you how my journey to regenerative brain health began. What I share with you I did not learn in medical school or in my hospital rotations during my internship and residency years. This was my own personal journey, supported by the wealth of knowledge of other doctors who opened up this path of knowledge in the fields of functional medicine and holistic medicine. I am grateful for what I have learned, because it has brought me back to resilient clarity of mind, and I want you to have the same opportunity and benefit from this approach to brain care.

My medical practice has deep ethical roots in the Hippocratic oath, which I took in 1994 when I graduated from medical school. This is an oath that all physicians take upon graduating. It states the following:

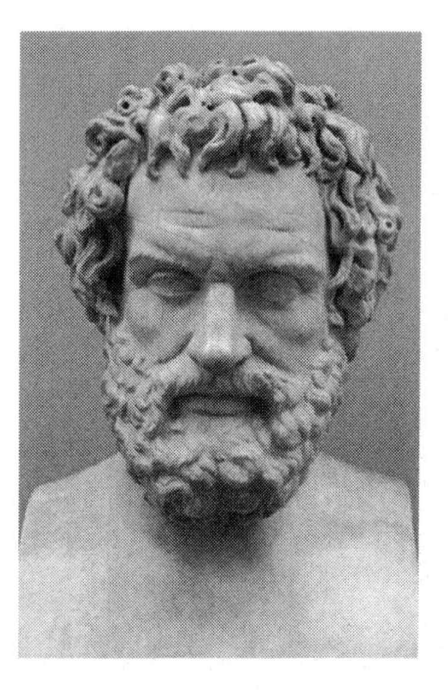

I do hereby affirm my loyalty to the profession I am about to enter. I will be mindful always of my great responsibility to preserve the health and the life of my patients, to retain their confidence and respect both as a physician and a friend who will guard their secrets with scrupulous honor and fidelity, to perform faithfully my professional duties, to employ only those recognized methods of treatment consistent with good judgment and with my skill and ability, keeping in mind always nature's laws and the body's inherent capacity for recovery.

Since taking that oath, I have attended over 150 conferences and spent thousands of hours learning and studying in order to better serve my patients. My patients' results and the information they have shared with me have culminated in both a wealth of knowledge and a solid body of clinical experience. My twenty-five-year romance with the body's intelligence has been a driving force in my career and medical practice; I have searched for a better understanding of the body's homeostatic mechanisms and marveled at the beauty of its structural scaffolding and physiological underpinnings. In keeping with the Hippocratic oath, I have sought to empower my patients with knowledge and practical resources—not to simply rely upon "quick-fix" drugs to treat a symptom, but rather to unearth the underlying cause. I also realize that most patients come to me because they seek to get well, once and for all. This is why I chose to make this book comprehensive and practical.

INTRODUCTION

Welcome to *Regenerate Your Brain.*

This book is my attempt to offer you the most pertinent and practical information you need to absorb in order to support your brain in the world of today and for the world we will face tomorrow. I am very glad that you have chosen to learn more about the many ways to optimize the health and performance of your brain—our body's most complex and important organ. As you will read in the pages that follow, I have a deep and personal interest in the health and regenerative capacity of the brain. My passion for brain health arose out of my own life experiences, and I am honored that I have an opportunity to share the fruits of my personal journey with you. It is my hope that this book will be a benefit to you and to those you love.

We are living in a time when the discoveries in neuroscience are exploding into the scene of our lives. I recall as a young girl on a clear summer night, looking up at the twinkling stars. I was both awestruck and stupefied as I contemplated the immensity of material form outside our earth's atmosphere. Part of me wanted to "scratch an itch" inside my brain and ponder the mind-boggling reality of the Milky Way and its stars that lie thousands of light years away, stars that we have discovered but will never be able to really know firsthand.

Now, decades later, I feel the same sense of awe that I felt as a little girl contemplating the cosmos when I consider the miracle of our human biology and the inner workings of the brain. Tending to our brain with wise medicine is perhaps the most important foundational health care decision we can make for our lives.

Attention Overload

The material world around me has changed dramatically since I spent those magical nights gazing at the heavens. The digital era was born, bringing with it a dizzying array of information and high-speed communication. Computer screens now convey writing in digital form instead of ink on paper. Smartphones and the internet have taken over as primary modalities of business communication. Gone are the days of handwritten letters, and absent are the subtle expressions of the eyes and the tonality of a voice in a business transaction that occurs in person, or even a "hello" via text. Emoticons have taken over the warm smile of a passerby. Clearly the speed and ease of access to information has logarithmically increased in recent years, with no signs of slowing down.

What is the cost of this?

Shauna Shapiro, PhD, author of *Good Morning, I Love You*, says, "We are exposed to forty gigabytes of information a day and one movie has three to four gigabytes, that's ten movies a day of information." Herbert A. Simon, American economist, political scientist, and cognitive psychologist declared this in 1971: "What information consumes is attention."

In this enlightening journey, I have felt a deep sense of urgency as I see the rapidity of changes in our modern world steamrolling ahead. In today's fast-paced modern world, a tragedy is occurring. It is silent and misunderstood. We are literally losing our minds! Our modern lifestyle is causing us to override a pace that would normally balance our brain and keep our nervous system in check. Our central nervous system—the ultimate part of our anatomy that controls our thoughts, actions, motivations, emotions, and physiology—is becoming unable to balance itself.

A few specifics illustrate the extent of this crisis:

- 44 percent of adults in the US between the ages of 75 and 84 have Alzheimer's.[1]
- Deaths from heart disease decreased 11 percent in 2018 while deaths from Alzheimer's increased 123 percent.[2]
- 26 percent of the US population is on one or more psychiatric medications.[3]
- Learning disabilities in children have increased 16 percent;[4] they occur in 1 out of 6 children, according to 2018 data from the Centers for Disease Control (CDC).
- CDC data from 2016 reveal that 9 percent of children between the ages 2 and 17 are diagnosed with attention deficit disorder.[5]

My Goal

My goal in writing this book is to keep you out of those statistics! As you will read in the pages ahead, the silent attack on our minds is rooted in the perils of pollution, pace, polypharmacy, and poor understanding.

This book offers you simple steps, tools, and resources to restore, repair, and regenerate your brain.

As I mentioned above, our brain is arguably the most complex and important organ in our body—*it really, really matters!* When I healed my own attention deficit disorder, the quality of my relationships deepened; I was able to follow through on and complete tasks in a timely manner and received job promotions; and my energy doubled, as I spent less energy spinning in my mind. I almost felt like I had stepped into my body as a different person, even though my underlying values and personality traits were the same. The truth is, when my brain started working better, everything in my life improved. Clear decisions came more rapidly, the energy it took to get things done dropped in half, and my anxiety disappeared. People entrusted in me more. I felt more appreciated in all my relationships and my sense of connectedness to my purpose grew. I felt capable of the life I was supposed to be leading rather than beleaguered by what felt like gravel in my shoes. Now I could sprint through tasks like a cheetah. I felt so good. Ultimately, I want to share this information so that other people can feel just as good.

Ironically, many of us know very little about this amazing organ that enables us "to know" in the first place.

Let me take you on a very short tour of the cosmos inside our skulls.

- Our brains comprise approximately 100 billion neurons.
- There are close to 10,000 synapses in every large neuron, each one firing 1,000 times a second.
- There are 100 million microtubules in each neuron. These microtubules connect the inside of each neuron to an outer matrix that lies outside the body's trillions of cells. Microtubules traverse along every muscle, bone, blood vessel, and organ. You can think of them as our internal internet, as they are literally an internal net allowing rapid exchange of information in every region of our body.
- The brain has two lobes. The right lobe is in charge of our visuospatial abilities, and the left lobe is in charge of speech and language. Together, they make up the cerebrum.
- Below the cerebrum is the cerebellum, which is in charge of our balance and muscle coordination, and all the cranial nerves, which are responsible for movement and for all our senses, including our eyes and eye muscles, as well as swallowing, hearing, smelling, tasting, and touching.

The brain stem connects the cerebrum to the cerebellum. Clearly, the way we think and the way our brains function shape every aspect of our lives. When we learn how to take care of our brains properly, implementing simple practical steps in our daily lives to support brain health, not only can we optimize our potential, but we can also avoid the nightmares of neurological illness. This book gives you simple and practical solutions to one of the most complex issues we face in our lives—the health of our brains.

If you are committed to improving the health of your brain and are ready to take the necessary steps to empower yourself, congratulations! You've chosen the right book. But this book is only a tool. Without your commitment and involvement, it will be of little value to you. For example, if your commitment level is 5 on a scale of 1 to 10 (with 10 being the highest), then you should put this book down now.

If instead you want real results, go inside yourself and assess your commitment level. *The higher your commitment, the higher your potential for real and lasting positive results.*

This book was written for people who are committed at the level of 10. It was written for people who, for example, are experiencing brain fog, poor focus, a lack of attentiveness, and moodiness. It was written for people who feel depressed or anxious, who feel their job performance is slipping, or who may be exhibiting some early signs of dementia. It was also written for people who have a family member or friend diagnosed with Parkinson's, a stroke, autism, or Alzheimer's. This book was designed for those loved ones while empowering you with tools to prevent such conditions from ever happening to you!

People Heal Themselves

But books don't heal people. People heal themselves. At the same time, I've noticed an incongruity between the expectations of my patients and the reality of the meticulous and often slow pace of their journey back to health. Many patients have become so accustomed to expecting a prescription pill to swallow and fix their problems immediately that they can't entertain the idea of a long-term practical plan. For some, the seemingly extraneous efforts of collecting urine samples at home, spitting into a tube for a saliva sample, going to the lab for blood work, and taking supplements twice a day seem like too much effort.

This book provides a road map to understand how to get from poor brain functioning to mental clarity and why each step matters.

My goal in writing this book has been to provide information about the most complex and least understood organ in our body, and to offer simple, practical, results-driven information for busy people who genuinely want to improve their brain health. As you will learn, there is no one-pill solution for healing your brain. In fact, a recent study reported that 234 out of 244 drug trials using the "one pill will fix it" model for Alzheimer's disease have failed.

Therefore, I'd like to explain in as concise a manner as I can why this complex organ of crucial significance in our lives deserves some committed care. I would like you not only to understand the why and how behind regenerative brain care but also to be able to make immediate changes to support your cognitive health. This means providing you not only with the theoretical and physiological explanations about the brain that I find fascinating, but also offering you practical tools such as lists of foods for your pantry and refrigerator, laboratory tests (labs) that offer meaningful results, and supplements to help boost your brain's functioning. I even offer the names of some smartphone apps I have created for you to use for meditation and other ways to enhance your brain health.

Optimal health is a daily practice. Exercising and eating healthy is not a new concept. We need to expand this concept to include our brain. Fortunately, caring for our brain can be simple and enjoyable, and can yield great benefits not just for our brain but our whole-body vitality.

When we turn our attention to our brain health, we say yes to every aspect of our lives.

How to Use This Book

As I stated earlier, this book is written as a practical guide for intelligent yet non-scientific and non-medically trained readers. It is organized for ease of use, detail of explanation, reference, and application by people who are truly committed to their brain health.

- **In Part One** (chapters 1 and 2), I offer my personal story, to provide you with the background and context for my personal and professional fascination with regenerating your brain. I also review the basic steps of this brain care program.
- **In Part Two** (chapters 3 through 9), I describe in greater detail the individual steps of regenerative brain care and how they fit together. I explain the physiology behind what helps your brain and also cite some of the research.
- **In Part Three** is a resources section that contains links to videos you can watch, other offerings of mine, retreat centers to attend, recipes to cook from, and people to contact for certain equipment or supplements.This guidebook is designed to give you a complete path for your own brain healing. I applied many of the things I write about in this book to my own journey of healing my brain. Many books out there describe the physiology behind neuroplasticity, offer certain intriguing case studies, and give you some good theory and research. However, few books are written for immediate practical application.

The truth is this: every 66 seconds another American over 65 develops dementia. I want to keep you out of those statistics!

This book is designed as both an information resource and a practical day-to-day guide. It doesn't have to be read from beginning to end in a linear order, though you may find this helpful. Feel free to jump to chapters or areas of interest. The key is to use it as a way to take meaningful steps on your journey to optimal brain health. If you find this book of value in this regard, I will have accomplished my mission.

If you have further questions—or if you would like to discuss how I may be of further support to you on your journey to optimal brain health—please don't hesitate to contact me through my website. Together we can take practical steps while marveling at this miraculous organ we call the brain.

Thank you,
Dr. Jacqueline
www.drjacqueline.com

PART ONE

"Optimal health includes operating out of the highest expression of our soul's purpose. The body intuitively wants to heal itself."

—Dr. Jacqueline Chan

1 | MY STORY

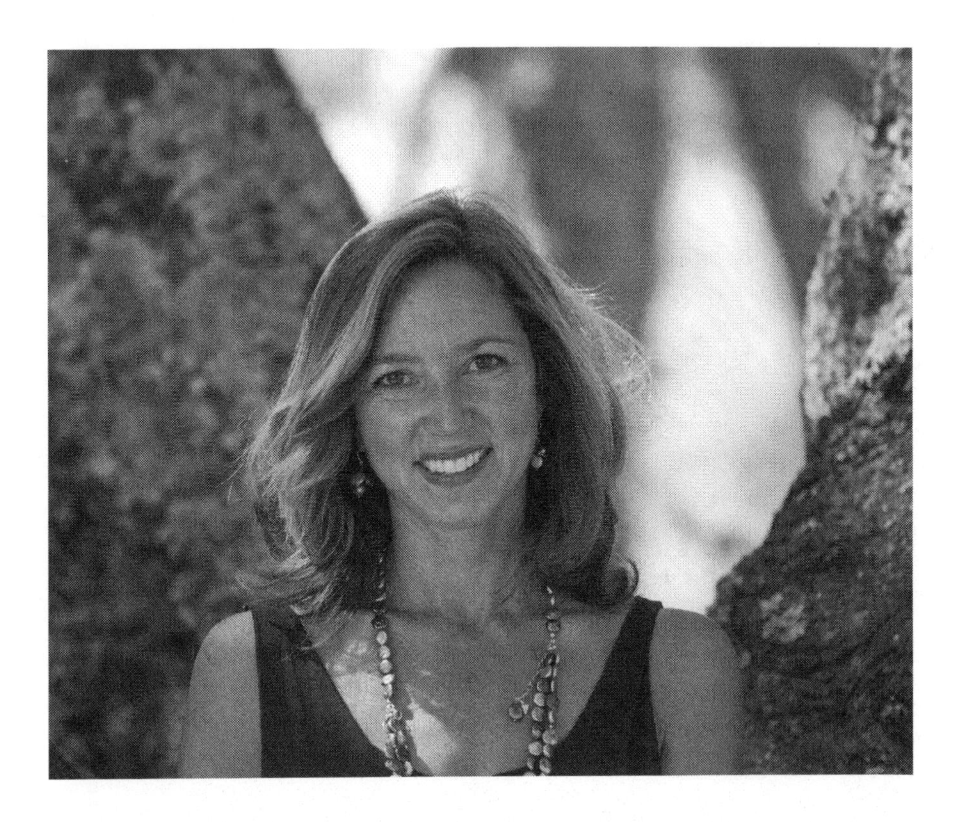

My life has exposed me to multiple different blessings and challenges that have resulted in an unusual, open-minded approach to science and healing. Although I spent a solid twenty years in Ohio with a mother who was a nurse and a stepfather who was an English professor, my life was far from that of a typical Midwestern American. Born in Galashiels, Scotland, and growing up in Edinburgh, I spent my early formative, school years wearing a tartan skirt and having tea parties. Meanwhile my mother was German and my father half-Spanish and half-Chinese. I traded the American family barbecue for multiple trips to Europe. And my cousins, aunts, and uncles lived in Germany, Spain, and Singapore. None of my blood was American. I am half-German, one-quarter Chinese and one-quarter Spanish. No one country or culture ever felt like home to me, until I was in a multicultural mix, such as the Bay Area of California, where I reside now. My career path has been a solid central structure in my life. My one true unending song of passion has been serving as a physician and healer.

In 1990, I was young, ambitious, eager, and wanting to serve. I had just completed my studies at Mount Holyoke College in Massachusetts, earning a liberal arts degree *magna cum laude* in philosophy. At this juncture, I decided to pursue a career as a physician.

The summer before entering medical school, I took an intensive organic chemistry class for my premed requirements. I also decided to work as a home health aide to beef up my medical school application. My granny has always had a special place in my heart, and since I love the elderly, it was only natural that I sought work in nursing homes and the private homes of the elderly. I had no idea that this early experience in my medical career would also introduce me to a terrible disease of the brain.

A Once-Brilliant Attorney's Nightmare Disease

One of my first patients—let's call her Gilda—lived in a gorgeous retirement home. She had been an attorney, while her husband had owned many of the office buildings in downtown Columbus, Ohio. When I first met Gilda, she came walking out of her bedroom wearing her bra on the outside of her dress. As she approached me, she took her purse, threw it at me, cussed at me, and began to cry.

This was an Alzheimer's picture, I later learned. This once-brilliant attorney who could cite statutes from memory could now not even remember the names of her children or husband when I pointed them out to her in photographs. She would get easily frustrated if I asked her questions about the past, sometimes even violently so, throwing a fork at me or walking away from me with great agitation. She kept wanting to "go home." But she *was* home. As my first Alzheimer's patient, she unwittingly introduced me to the nightmare of what can happen when our brains become diseased. I could only imagine how devastating it was for her daughter and son to visit her and go unrecognized. This is a disease that leads to crippling consequences for millions of people. Little did I know then that I would actually have something to offer Gilda years later, if she were still alive today—something that could have helped regenerate her brain health.

Bicycle Accident in Ireland

My exposure to the fragilities of the brain did not end with Alzheimer's. Fortunately, I was accepted into my top choice of medical schools and graduated in the top ten of my class. Yet I was haunted by my experience with Gilda and all the other elderly in similar situations, and I remained keenly interested in neuroscience and the health of the brain. It wasn't until I was in my thirties that I realized that an event that happened when I was a young teenager had created a scary insult to my brain, which affected me at a very personal level. When I was fourteen years old, I had had a serious accident while on a bike tour with my family in Ireland. This was at a time before bicycle helmets were in style. After falling from my racing bike at 35 mph, I hit my head on the pavement and suffered a severe brain concussion. I was kept in the hospital for six days and afterwards was still having trouble remembering my name or how to walk. Prior to the accident I had been a 4.0 GPA student. After the hospital discharge, I had to work a lot harder to keep making good grades. My lessons in brain health were only just beginning.

Fast-forward to my late thirties. I decided to live out my dream by moving from Ohio to California. I was engaged to be married and I felt the world was my oyster. Although I lived in an idyllic setting in a small artistic community overlooking the Pacific Ocean, the changes rocked me. Everything was new, and I found myself getting easily overwhelmed, often tearful. A patient gave me a book on the six types of attention deficit disorder (ADD) by Daniel Amen, MD. For the first time, I read that trauma to the area of my brain that was injured in the bicycle accident could cause ADD. As I read about all the symptoms of ADD, I realized to my own embarrassment that *I had almost all of them!* My fiancé said 90 percent of our relationship problems were related to my ADD symptoms. For example, I would think I'd heard him say something when I hadn't really captured it, or I would forget things he told me.

In the end my fiancé and I broke up, and I can't help but think that my ADD was a significant factor. I even measured my brain chemistry through a urine test (by measuring my neurotransmitters), which revealed I had a low serotonin level, a finding often correlating with a brain concussion. Even though I was living my dream in a gorgeous home by the ocean, with plenty of time off and in a new romantic relationship, my brain chemistry was the same as that of someone who is depressed. Seeking a cure, I tried the standard allopathic prescription for ADD—a stimulant—and I couldn't sleep for two days. Surely, this medication was not the solution. As you will read later in this book, I eventually discovered some key supplements that helped my ADD based on my brain's unique chemistry. And I felt radically better!

A Walk in the Woods

Moving from Ohio to Muir Beach, California, was a dream come true for me. I felt as though the heavens had sent a ray of light into my life, bringing me incredible outdoor beauty only five minutes from my front

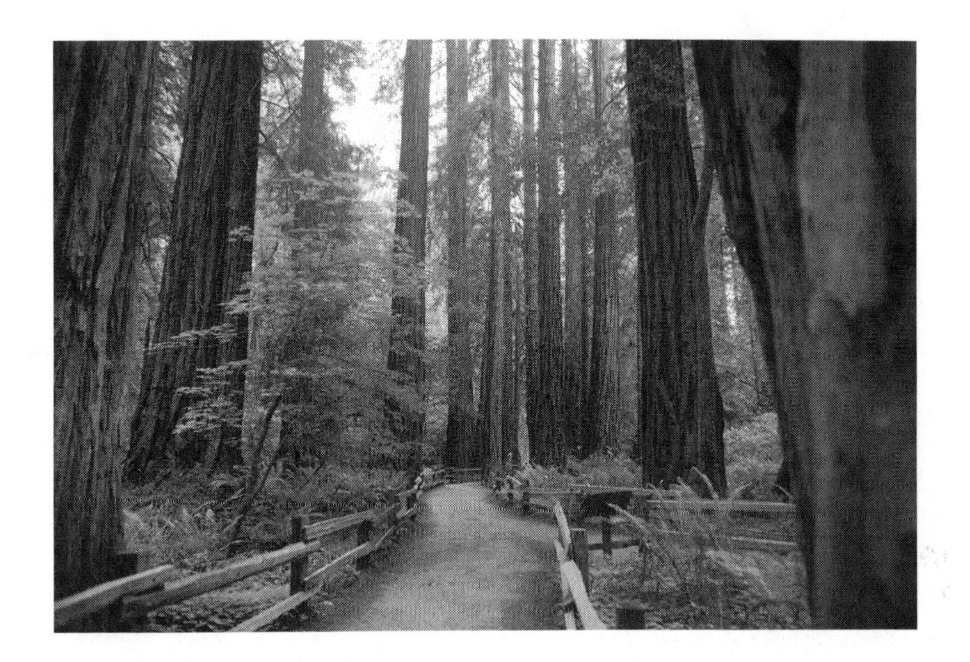

door. I never took it for granted. My favorite grove in Muir Woods is called Cathedral Grove. You are asked to be silent as you walk through the forest of tall glorious trees that have been around since before the time of Christopher Columbus.

However, sometimes life gifts us with a grain of sand when our lives are running the most smoothly. What happened next was a downward twist in my path of good fortune. As hard as it was, crippling me for about one year, I would not have written this book if it hadn't happened, and there was nothing I could have done to stop it from happening.

While I was adjusting to my new single life in California, I would often walk in the redwood forest, for refueling and inspiration. One day while hiking in the gorgeous redwood groves of Muir Woods, I rested my head against the trunk of a tree and a nymph tick climbed into my ponytail. While I was driving home, it fell onto my forearm.

There were many deer in the woods, and I knew to watch out for deer ticks. But this tick was tiny, about the size of the tip of a ballpoint pen, and I certainly never felt it in my ponytail. It was identified as a nymph tick, known to be associated with three infections: *Borrelia*, *Bartonella*, and *Babesia*.

Ironically, I was working with a nationally known Lyme disease expert at the time, because Lyme disease had become an epidemic in California, and many of my patients had come to me with a multitude of symptoms related to Lyme disease that had gone undiagnosed. Having seen the nymph tick on my arm, I took antibiotics for three weeks as a preventive measure and exhibited no symptoms; I felt fine. Yet three months later, I began to need a second cup of coffee at noon to make it through the day. I noticed that by 8:00 p.m. I was ready to go to bed, and I had an ongoing mild sore throat and fever. I just thought I had a bit of a cold.

Yet another month passed, and I began to have a Parkinson's-like tremor in my left hand as well as a motor tic in my face.

This got my attention.

I went to a close colleague and he diagnosed me with Lyme disease, babesiosis and bartonellosis infection. After six weeks of triple antibiotics, I was significantly better, but my brain speed was lagging. I felt as though I was operating at half throttle. I took a vacation, but the slowness in my brain did not improve. I became agitated more easily by interruptions. My memory was so challenged that I became the Post-it note queen—I even had Post-it notes for my other Post-it notes! One day I got lost four times driving to the airport. As you might imagine, this level of functioning was totally unacceptable to me.

What ensued was a fascinating journey back to full health. I learned during this time that the infection from the tick bite had gone to the part of my brain that was scarred from the bicycle fall at age fourteen.

After one year of treatment with three different antibiotics, a number of powerful herbal formulas, immune system boosting IVs, and hyperbaric oxygen therapy, I felt like I got my brain back! In fact, I could think sixteen times faster than ever before. I had a voracious appetite to learn again. I went from working two days a week back to five days a week and from needing ten hours of sleep back to seven hours. I became happy again. My bouts of crying and feeling overwhelmed stopped.

Later in this book, I'll share with you one of the healing therapies I've discovered. After using this therapy, I experienced a flashback to the bicycle fall years earlier. It was at that point that I knew my brain scar was being healed!

A Dizzying Experience

After recovering from the bicycle accident and the tick bite, I thought my brain journey was over. But I was wrong. Just over two years before writing this book, I had the scariest brain event ever. It was December 2016, very close to Christmas, when I began to have dizzy spells. While sitting at my desk, I felt as though the whole table was tipping and I was about to fall off my chair. This sensation was very strong.

Around this time, I had a strong premonition—*something was wrong with a family member of mine … horribly wrong.* My dad was living in Spain at the time and I communicated with him about once a month via Skype. He was in tip-top shape, still working at the age of seventy-nine. I had a strong feeling in my gut that something was wrong with him and that my dizziness was somehow linked to his illness.

I reached out to his Spanish wife and asked, "Is Dad in the hospital?" to which she responded, "Who told you?"

I said, "No one. I just felt something was really wrong."

She replied, "Yes, he's been in the hospital two days and didn't want me to say anything to you yet."

As I pondered my father's long-distance hospitalization, my dizziness persisted. I thought perhaps it was because my blood sugar was down, but I noticed the dizziness would happen even after a full meal. I wondered if it was work-related stress, but it also happened when I was just standing in the kitchen wearing my bathrobe and drinking tea.

I decided to go to a neurologist. She discovered that my blood pressure was 200/130, high enough to cause a stroke. I was shocked! As a petite athletic woman, I had had ideal blood pressure of 90/60 most of my life and 110/70 at the highest. My neurological reflexes indicated that I might be having a ministroke. I immediately took aspirin, did a battery of tests, and bought a blood pressure cuff to use at home. That very day I opened my email to share with my dad that I had high blood pressure, only to find that he had just emailed me to share that he had been diagnosed with prostate cancer. The coincidence of us both having a health crisis almost on the same day was impossible for me to dismiss. While this coincidence puzzled me and didn't make scientific sense, it did make sense intuitively. Thankfully, within one week my dizziness miraculously ended and my blood pressure normalized.

Then, while I was writing this book in May 2018, I also suffered a head injury from a car accident. I became very dizzy once again, even though my blood pressure was now completely normal. I had a hard time focusing for four months. Yet once again, with the help of the therapies I mention in this book, I became mentally sharp and clear again.

These experiences—and many, many more—have contributed to my decision and desire to write a brain health guidebook that would be useful for others. I have often wondered how my experience might have been different if I had had a guidebook such as this one at the time when I was in the midst of these mysterious and debilitating conditions of my body's most important organ. In writing this book, it is my sincere hope and desire to share with you what I did to regenerate my brain, and in so doing to give you a complete path for your own brain health and healing.

2 | THE SOLUTION

The discovery that my brain may have a medical problem was embarrassing for me—embarrassing, scary, and hard to face. After all, it was my excellent academic performance in high school and college that had gotten me into medical school. The complexity of medicine requires not only caring for the suffering of other humans but also having a clear logical mind to go through the differential diagnosis of a patient, come up with an effective treatment plan based on the accurate application of remedies, and stay on top of the latest medical literature, evolving lab work, and administrative documentation.

Just as I cared about how other people suffered, I needed to realize that I too was actually suffering. I found spending time on my computer's electronic screens particularly stressful; the multiple insults to my brain had affected an aspect of my visual tracts, causing this great amount of stress. I knew I couldn't address my problems until I admitted to myself that I had problems and then committed to addressing them.

My kind of suffering wasn't obvious to an outsider in the same way a broken bone or a limp or a rash would be. My suffering felt more like overwhelm, agitation, feeling empty and sad for no reason, and experiencing a mind that kept racing. These feelings I learned later weren't because of a weakness in my character or a flaw in my consciousness—they were actually occurring because my brain was malfunctioning. It felt as though having a malfunctioning brain made it harder for me to fully express who I truly am and to behave in a reliable manner. I had perfect attendance in high school growing up, and yet I struggled to be on time as my ADD worsened. It was as if my brain couldn't understand "clock time."

The good news was that there was nothing wrong with *me*, the person; it was my *physical brain* that needed the help. This realization proved to be a powerful force in my healing, and it freed me to seek medical help without the fear, stigma, or embarrassment that is so often associated with brain-related illnesses.

In my medical practice over many years, I have observed brain problems of many kinds showing up in my patients. Following are a number of such medical diagnoses:

Anxiety

Asperger's

Attention deficit disorder

Autism

Bipolar disease

Dementia

Depression

Obsessive-compulsive disorder

Parkinson's

Other conditions which aren't actually diseases but still indicate that the brain could use some help are these:

Brain fog

Chronic stress

Difficulty focusing

Inattentiveness

Insomnia

Irritability

Memory loss

If you have—or think you may have—one of the above conditions, you may feel upset or ashamed, but you should know that you are not alone. Brain disorders are actually a silent epidemic in today's America. These statistics were presented by the National Alliance on Mental Health in 2015:

- One out of five Americans experiences a mental illness some time in their life.
- 42 million Americans (18.1 percent) experience anxiety.
- Depression is the leading cause of disability worldwide and a major contributor to the global burden of disease.
- Half of all chronic mental illnesses begin by age fourteen and the other half by age twenty-four.

Even if you go through life unbrushed by mental illness, your risk of developing Alzheimer's disease is as high as 30 percent of adults, according to CDC 2018 data.

Although these statistics are pretty grim, if we pay attention to our brain health early on, we can prevent some of these occurrences. Current research shows that cognitive decline can begin ten to twenty years before an actual diagnosis (in the case of Alzheimer's, for example). Fortunately, new labs are beginning to reveal the physiological shifts that occur years before a diagnosis of Alzheimer's disease can be made.

Traditionally, brilliant scientists and pharmacists try to find a secret pill to fix the issue. For the brain, however, one has to look beyond

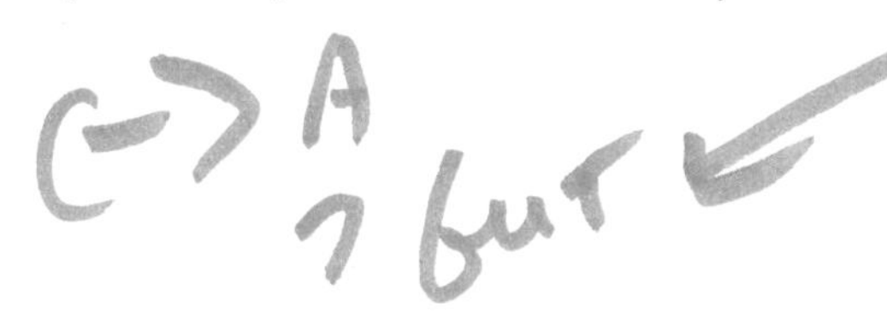

pharmaceuticals for the answer. No single drug has been found to stop or even slow the progression of Alzheimer's, and drugs have only had modest effects on symptoms. "In the past decade alone, hundreds of clinical trials have been conducted for Alzheimer's, without success, at an aggregate cost of over $1 billion," said Dale Bredesen, MD, researcher at the Buck Institute, an independent biomedical institute that researches aging and age-related disease. The mission of the Buck Institute is to extend the healthy years of life.

The truth is that the brain is too complex for a single drug agent to solve the problem. If you or someone you love suffers from a brain-related health issue, there is good news: *You are not alone.* The even better news is that **your brain can heal and even regenerate itself!** Thanks to a tremendous number of breakthroughs in neuroscience, there are many solutions now available that can help you maximize your brain health.

As an example of just how adaptive the brain is, it has been observed that infants who are born with one brain hemisphere missing generally grow up with normal brain function. In fact, an article in *National Geographic*'s April 2019 issue titled "Your Brain: 100 Things You Never Knew" (page 31) cites a case history exemplifying this neuroplasticity in a man from Massachusetts named Jonathan Keleher. As a child, Keleher was slow to walk and talk, but not until he was five did a brain scan reveal the problem: the boy completely lacked a cerebellum. The little structure at the back of the brain holds 50 percent of the brain's neurons. It controls vital functions: balance, posture, physical skills, and some language learning, among other things. Adults with damage to the cerebellum can be severely impaired or even die, and yet Keleher did learn to walk, falling and getting up and falling again. He learned to speak and grew up to hold a job and live a relatively normal life. Keleher's case, and others like it, show brain scientists just how "plastic" the young brain can be when the need arises.

Depending upon the circumstances, a person with brain health concerns may need to work with a physician for some of the recovery process. At the same time, there are now many easy, safe, and practical steps we can take in our everyday life.

Supporting your brain is perhaps one of the most important commitments you can make in your life. Learn to care for it with the latest science. I have designed the Regenerate Your Brain Program to support the optimization of your brain's cognitive performance and health, based on the latest scientific research. I focus on underlying causes for concern, rather than simply treating symptoms. The Program is based upon the discovery that the brain is a dynamic organ with the inherent ability to not only maintain itself but also to improve its functioning well into old age.

My brain care approach is adapted in part from the Mind Diet, a treatment approach used by UCLA and the Buck Institute Research on Aging, designed by Dale Bredesen, MD. In Dr. Bredesen's book, *The End of Alzheimer's*, he reports that with the approaches I'm about to outline, he helped reverse memory loss in 90 percent of his patients.

The Regenerate Your Brain Program expands upon the original Mind Diet concepts. It also include additional discoveries I have made over the years based upon my knowledge of osteopathic medicine in the cranial field, over twenty years of experience in functional medicine, and certification as a hyperbaric physician.

Osteopathic medicine is a whole-person approach to integrative medical care, recognized as a pioneering force in wellness medicine dating back to the early efforts of Andrew Taylor Still, MD, DO, in the 1870s. Guided by training that identifies the musculoskeletal system as a key element of health, we doctors of osteopathy use hands-on osteopathic manipulative treatment (OMT) to focus on your body's interconnected system of nerves, muscles, and bones. OMT is typically used to treat various sources of muscle and joint pain and conditions such as carpal tunnel syndrome. Additionally, it can be used to treat asthma, sinus disorders, migraines, and menstrual pain—often all without medications or more invasive medical procedures.

Osteopathy in the cranial field focuses more specifically on the skull, brain, and spinal cord. With skilled training and thousands of hours of practice, such as I have had, the motion and position of the twenty-three bones in the skull can be felt. Dural strains (strains within the membranes inside the skull) can be discerned and the position of the brain itself can be felt. I feel for things like whether the brain has slowed its motion, or whether the brain's pulsations are lopsided so that one hemisphere or lobe is limping along. I check whether the neurons are trembling, as if in reaction to trauma. I feel whether the sutures in the cranial bones are compressed. I feel whether the critical ganglion of the sympathetic and parasympathetic nervous system is damaged or on hyper mode. Being able to view the brain as an organ that can be helped through hands-on cranial osteopathic manipulation adds profound benefits to the healing of the brain.

The term *functional medicine* refers to the determination of how and why illness occurs, and it restores health by addressing the root causes of disease for each individual.

Hyperbaric oxygen certification involves passing an examination on the basic tenets of how hyperbaric oxygen physiologically assists in healing. Hyperbaric oxygen therapy (HBOT) consists of a person entering a chamber in which they are exposed to 100 percent medical-grade oxygen under pressure. I will discuss how HBOT helps in healing the brain in chapter 8, "Boosting Your Mitochondria."

Dr. Jacqueline Chan's Regenerate Your Brain Program

I break down the principles of regenerative brain care into seven major components to aid in simplification. These seven components are outlined below.

1. *Nourishing Your Brain*

Chapter 3, "Nourishing Your Brain," includes a dietary plan for brain performance based on years of research. We will look at how your brain functions with components such as fats, amino acids, and superfoods like turmeric, blueberries, and coffee. Cutting-edge lab work of your blood chemistry can reveal guideposts for the crucial vitamins and minerals missing in your nutrition. Optimal dietary choices create a powerful diet for your brain.

2. *Balancing Healthy Hormones*

In Chapter 4, "Balancing Healthy Hormones," we will look at how hormones influence our mood and our mental and physical behavior, by elucidating the roles of neurotransmitters, adrenal hormones, sex hormones, thyroid hormones, insulin, and melatonin, as well as bioidentical hormones. You will learn how to improve your energy and sleep, as well as balance difficult emotions such as anxiety, depression, anger, irritability, or addiction through the use of your diet and herbal plant medicine. I describe which lab work will assess your hormone levels.

3. *Healing the Gut-Brain Axis*

Chapter 5, "Healing Leaky Gut and Leaky Brain," teaches the causes of "leaky gut" and the functions of your *microbiome*—the body of bacteria inside your gut. It also explains what foods to eat and which ones to avoid in order to heal your gut. Get a head start with powerful nutrients that can speed up the healing of your gut.

4. *Cooling Brain Inflammation*

Chapter 6 identifies the things that cause inflammation in the brain. Read about nutritional and herbal supplementation proven to lower inflammation, detoxify, support genetic pathways, increase neuroplasticity, and optimize brain chemistry. I explain the importance of including cranial osteopathy for improving lymphatic drainage and enhancing the circulation of blood flow as well as cerebrospinal fluid flow to the brain. Cranial osteopathy results in increased delivery of oxygen and nutrients to damaged tissues. As well, it enhances the removal of carbon dioxide and other waste products of metabolism. We will explore what's possible through cranial osteopathic manipulation and exercises to release the tension in the vagus nerve. The vagus nerve is the longest of the twelve cranial nerves. It emerges from the brain to interface with the heart, lungs, and digestive tract and to innervate the heartbeat, respiratory rate, and peristaltic motion of the digestive tract.

5. *Eliminating Toxins and Detoxifying*

In chapter 7, we will identify toxins and learn how to avoid further toxin exposure. I will explain how mercury; Bisphenol A (BPA), from plastic; and glyphosate, from foods that have undergone genetic modification (GMOs), cause harm. I include a basic plan for detoxification.

6. *Boosting Your Mitochondria*

In chapter 8, I answer the question of where energy comes from in the body, and I reveal the power of certain exercises to boost your mitochondria, the energy-making factories in your body. We also take a look at what causes oxidative stress, which lowers your energy, and the true facts of aging. I will reveal in this chapter the neuro-nutrients that will boost your brain power, and I will explain the unique therapy of using medical-grade hyperbaric oxygen to nourish the mitochondria of the brain, create new blood vessels, and increase stem cell production to heal brain trauma.

7. *Soothing Your Mind*

Chapter 9 focuses on sleep and deep rest, which are crucial to optimal brain health. I give you some solid good-sleep practices to implement.

8. *Building New Neural Pathways*

Lastly, in Chapter 10 you will learn about the entire living matrix of a human body as a simultaneously mechanical, vibrational, energetic, electronic, and informational network. I discuss the importance of coherence as a healing force and how to increase your own coherence through your thoughts as well as other nature based practices such as forest bathing or pet therapy to help build new neural pathways.

You will learn an invisible yet valid component of our anatomy—the biofield. I will expose a rarely discussed aspect that affects our brain—electrical energy—and tell you what to do about it. This section of the book covers emotional and psychological influences such as trauma and adverse childhood events.

In chapter 10, I demonstrate how to lay down new neural pathways through regenerative practices, helping you to redesign your central nervous system. You will learn ways to sculpt your brain through your thoughts, journaling, and body awareness exercises. Finally, I discuss the pros and cons of technology, sharing with you two evidence-based types of technology for your everyday use that aid in clarity, memory building, and lowered stress.

The brain is an infinitely complex, sensitive, and crucial organ. We need it for so many vital life functions, including regulating our mood, making life-defining decisions, performing effectively at work, maintaining positive healthy relationships, and functioning well overall. In the Regenerate Your Brain Program, I want to provide you with everything I can to help you prevent dementia, reverse cognitive decline, enhance your mood and focus, and achieve peak performance.

While the Regenerate Your Brain Program offers great potential to achieve these goals, it doesn't run on autopilot. Far from it. Success will require your commitment to devote additional time to exercising, preparing healthy meals, organizing supplements, getting labs done, and coming to weekly or semi-monthly appointments for eight weeks. You can achieve full brain health if your commitment level is a 10! My staff and I are here to support you to do that and will match your level of commitment with our 100 percent dedication.

PART TWO

"All of these benefits I describe in this book don't just affect our brain cells. They're benefits are widespread throughout the entire body. "

—Dr. Jacqueline Chan

3 | NOURISHING YOUR BRAIN

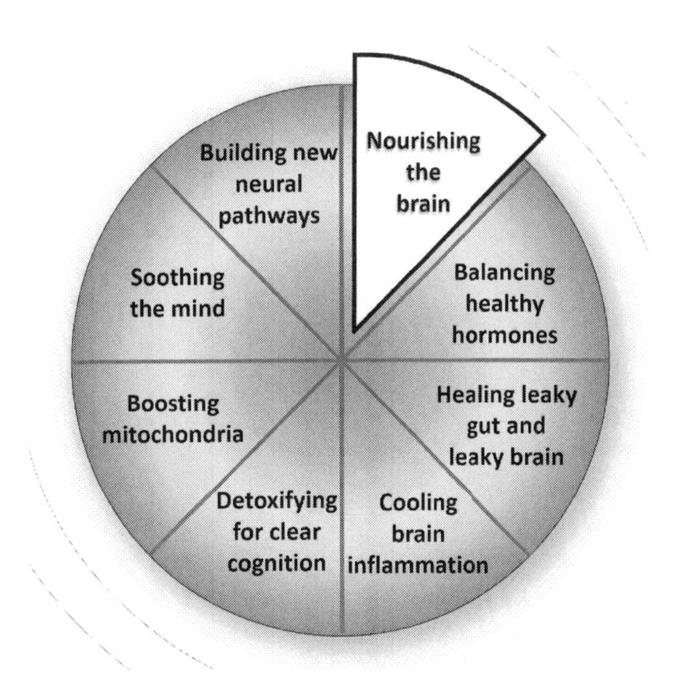

If we want to have healthy brains, we need to nourish our bodies with the right raw materials for building our brain chemistry, our cell membranes, and the nerves themselves. The optimal ingredients for brain health include these:

Essential fats

Fresh fruits and vegetables, and complex carbohydrates

Key amino acids from protein

Vitamins and minerals

These ingredients come from a diet of real, whole, local, fresh, unadulterated, unprocessed foods that are free of added chemicals, hormones, and antibiotics. I strongly advocate supporting this diet with essential vitamin and mineral supplements to ensure that you are getting all the raw materials your body and brain need for optimal function.

Fats and Your Brain

Few of us have ever actually seen, felt, or held a brain. When we think of the brain as a solid organ, the closest reference to it may be from the movie *Frankenstein*. If you actually could hold and touch a brain, you would realize it feels a lot like Jell-O with a bit more density to it. That's because approximately 60 percent of our brain is composed of fat. These fats are obtained in the form of fatty acids from the foods we eat, and they are among the most crucial molecules for maintaining your brain's integrity and performance ability. Just as rubber insulation is wrapped around the electrical wires for all our electrical appliances, so the fat in our brains helps to insulate the electrical signals

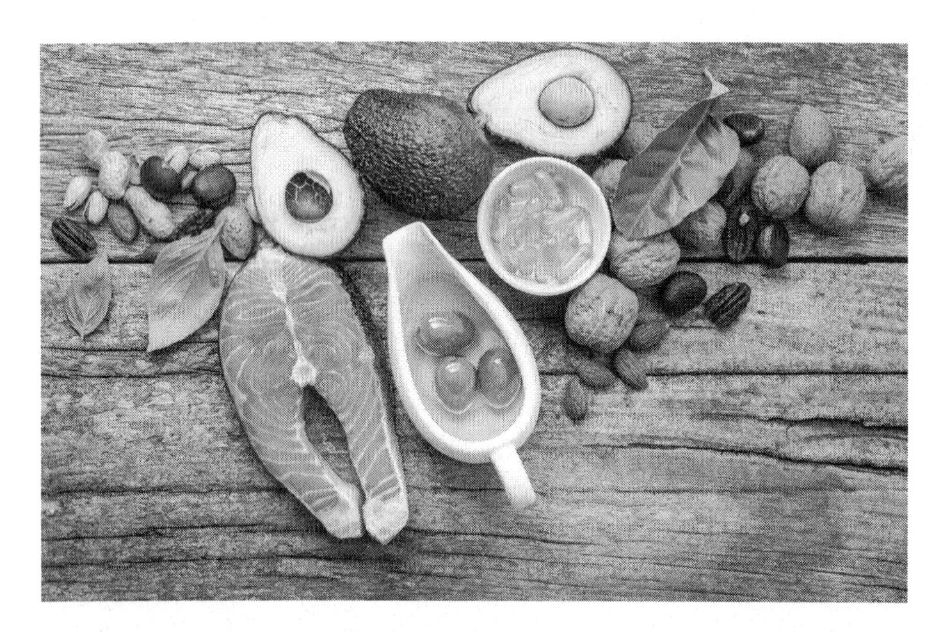

sent and received by our neurons to ensure that the signals are correctly transmitted.

The most important fats for a healthy brain are omega-3 fatty acids. Omega-3s are referred to as *essential fatty acids*. Because our bodies can't make them, they must be obtained from our diet. There are three types of omega-3s:

Alpha-linoleic acid (ALA)

Eicosapentaenoic acid (EPA)

Docosahexaenoic acid (DHA)

DHA represents 97 percent of all the omega-3 fats in the brain.[6] Optimal levels of DHA can reduce your risk of dementia, anxiety, and depression.

Omega-3s have anti-inflammatory effects that have been shown to protect the heart and to reduce rates of depression, dementia, obesity, diabetes, metabolic syndrome, autoimmune disease, kidney disorders, and even cancer.

Inadequate levels of omega-3s in our diet have been shown to be linked to many physical and mental disorders, including attention deficit hyperactivity disorder (ADHD), bipolar disease, dyslexia, depression, anxiety, and schizophrenia.

A great deal of scientific data supports this, including an impressive article titled "The Role of Omega-3 Fatty Acids in the Treatment of Depressive Disorders: A Comprehensive Meta-Analysis of Randomized Clinical Trials," which is a meta-analysis of nineteen trials, published in the May 7, 2014, edition of *PLOS One*, available in the US National Library of Medicine National Institutes of Health.[7]

Here is a sample of research on omega-3 fatty acids:

1. A meta-analysis published last year of the combined test data of over one million subjects found that the highest consumption of omega-3s from fish oil was associated with a 15 percent

reduction in the risk of dying from any cause compared with the lowest category. The study also found a 7 percent reduction in the overall risk of dying for each additional 200 mg of fish oil consumed per day.[8]

2. In a study of adults with mild cognitive impairment (which often precedes dementia), a daily supplement of 720 mg EPA plus 480 mg DHA (key forms of omega-3 fats) improved basic cognitive amplitude, speed of perception, and working memory compared with people receiving a placebo.[9]
3. One study evaluated the impact of omega-3s on women with major depression associated with menopause. After eight weeks of taking 930 mg EPA plus 750 mg DHA daily, the average standardized depression score fell by 56 percent.[10]
4. Seniors with higher levels of DHA are 47 percent less likely to develop dementia.[11]

If there were a pharmaceutical drug that could lower dementia rates by 47 percent and depression by 56 percent, it would be prescribed by every doctor! Yet few physicians think of the importance of omega-3 fatty acids.

High quality omega-3 fatty acids are available from certain classes of foods, both plant-based and animal-based. Plant-based omega-3s come from seeds and nuts, in the form of ALA: in walnuts, hempseed, flaxseed, and chia. If you choose to eat flaxseed and hempseed, the best way is to use a coffee grinder to grind them into a powder; otherwise they pass through the digestive tract whole and unabsorbed because the seeds are so small. When you grind the seeds, you get their lignans and fiber. You can sprinkle this seed powder as a condiment on your salads, stir-fry it with vegetables, mix it in with the batter of baked goods, or include it in cereal or porridge to add a nice nutty flavor.

Animal-based omega-3 fatty acids come predominantly from wild fish.

At a minimum, we need to ingest 1,000 mg of omega-3 fatty acids a day, but levels of 2,000 to 4,000 mg a day are recommended in situations that involve brain trauma, heart disease, and cognitive decline.

The best food sources for omega-3 are as follows:

- **Fish:** (see the resources section for a more comprehensive list)
  mackerel (7,000 mg per 8 oz.)
  herring (5,700 mg per 8 oz.)
  wild salmon (1,700 mg per 3 oz.)
  tuna (1,400 mg per 3 oz.)
  white fish (1,400 mg per 3 oz.)
  sardines (1,400 mg per 3.75-oz. can)
  anchovies (1,000 mg per 2-oz. can)
  The smaller fish have less mercury.
- **Walnuts:** seven walnuts contain about 2,500 mg.
- **Chia seeds:** one tbsp. contains about 2,500 mg.
- **Ground flaxseed:** one tbsp. contains about 1,500 mg.
- **Ground hempseeds:** one tbsp. contains about 1,000 mg.
- **Egg yolks:** one egg yolk contains about 225 mg.
- **Beans:** tofu, which is made from soybeans, has over 32 mg of DHA per 14 oz.; navy beans have 1,190 mg per cup.
- **Spinach, brussels sprouts, kale, and watercress:** these have about 350 mg per half cup, once cooked.

As mentioned above, the cells of our brains are made up mostly of fat; approximately 97 percent of each cell consists of DHA, an important type of omega-3. In addition, every cell membrane in your brain and body is made up of omega-3 fats. This is important, because if your cell membranes contain a healthy amount of omega-3s, your brain and body will function optimally. In particular, when the receptor sites in the cell membranes function well, the signaling that occurs within the cell will be optimal. In addition to improving signaling, good quality omega-3s and other healthful fatty acids ensure that cell membranes remain elastic instead of becoming stiff and brittle as we age. Elastic cell membranes improve our brain cells' ability to receive and send biochemical messages in a clear and distinct way. If our cell membranes aren't highly functional, the speed of communication of biochemical messages slows down.

What else do healthy omega-3 fats do for our brains aside from building cells and cell membranes? They also help reduce inflammation, balance blood sugar, and increase the activity of a key brain molecule called *brain-derived nerve factor* (BDNF), which stimulates new cell growth and increases cell connections. I describe this further in the later chapters of this book.

Amino Acids

Now that you understand that most of the brain is made of fat, you are probably wondering what comprises the other part of the brain. Aside from fat, your brain is specifically made up of the amino acid building blocks that get transformed into neurotransmitters. These are messenger molecules that are produced by nerve cells to communicate and control almost every function of your body. I will cover the neurotransmitters in detail in chapter 4, "Balancing Healthy Hormones." The neurotransmitters are chemical messengers that act a little like the accelerator and brake in your car—they stimulate you or calm you down. The key to being a happy, healthy, focused, and attentive human being is a balance between the excitation and tranquil rest that your nervous system modulates. These neurotransmitters are built from the proteins you get in your diet, specifically from the eight essential amino acids that you must get from the foods you eat. You must have these eight amino acids in your diet in order to make your neurotransmitters: isoleucine,

leucine, lysine, methionine, phenylalanine, threonine, tryptophan, and valine. All sources of animal protein, such as meat, fish, and chicken, give you these eight amino acids. If you are eating mostly vegetables on a vegetarian diet, you may be lacking these amino acids. Therefore, it's important to supplement with a source of protein, such as brown rice protein or pea protein. I provide medical food drinks that have all these proteins in them in the resources section at the back of the book.

Serotonin is a key neurotransmitter. The *Broken Brain* video series by Mark Hyman, MD, reveals this scary truth:

> *SSRIS, which are the most frequently prescribed antidepressants, are designed to make more serotonin available in your body. The way they do that is by blocking the reuptake of this neurotransmitter once it's been used.*

Dr. Hyman goes on to elucidate why antidepressants ultimately fail us. Let me explain. After serotonin binds to cells and delivers its message of happiness, it's exhausted. It flows away from the cells and into your detoxification system to be recycled and disposed. This is what is called *reuptake*. By blocking this process, those medicines essentially beat your poor serotonin as though it were a dead horse. They ask one neurotransmitter to do more and more work without replenishing your actual serotonin levels. This approach is completely backward. It works against our biochemistry. More importantly it never even approaches the question that is begging to be asked: "Why is your serotonin level low in the first place?"

There may be many reasons, as you will discover from reading this book, and they are related to nutritional deficiencies, high levels of stress, inflammation, toxins, dysregulation, and genetic predispositions.

If you are a vegetarian, consider adding 5-hydroxytryptophan (5-HTP), 100 to 200 mg once or twice a day away from food, to increase your serotonin production. Please only do this with caution and a physician's assistance if you are concomitantly taking a psychiatric medication.

Good Carbohydrates and Rainbow Colors

Whole plants provide healthy carbohydrates for our body and brain. Because the brain especially feeds on glucose, that glucose should ideally come from complex carbohydrates derived from plant-based foods. Healthy glucose is slowly released from the complex structure of plants, which are also the source of fiber and phytonutrients that protect you from a host of diseases. Phytonutrients are responsible for the rainbow colors found in fruits and vegetables, such as the red in cherries; the blue in blueberries; the orange in squash, oranges, and carrots; and the dark green in spinach. These brightly colored phytonutrients defend our cells by helping maintain deoxyribonucleic acid (DNA) stability from damage caused by oxidative stress. Strive to eat at least ten different foods a day, with five to nine servings of vegetables and two to four servings of fruits.

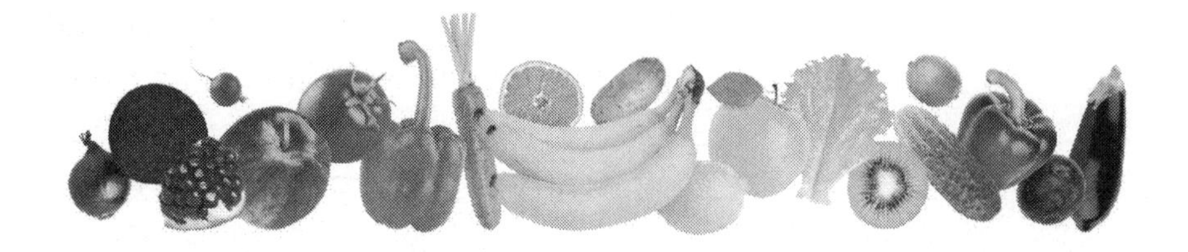

Turmeric

Turmeric plants are bright orange in color. They look like ginger root. It's the turmeric in curry that makes curry yellow. This color is a polyphenol called curcumin. It acts as a micronutrient with antioxidant activity. Turmeric, also called curcumin, has been popular in India for five thousand years. Curcumin may help aging blood vessels to relax and increase blood flow to the brain.

Turmeric can be enjoyed by adding it to your cooking as a sauce or in curries. It's best absorbed with some black pepper and healthy fats, such as ghee or butter.

An optimal way to absorb the curcuminoids in turmeric is to take it in the patented supplement form, which increases its bioavailability. At a dose of 2 gm curcumin alone, serum levels were either undetectable or very low in human volunteers. But curcumin administered with piperine (the chief active ingredient of pepper) produced much higher serum concentrations with a 2000 percent increase in bioavailability. I like to use Xymogen's combined fish oil and curcumin product. One capsule twice a day optimizes the benefits of fish oil and curcumin together.

Research has demonstrated that curcumin has antioxidant activity, is an immune cell modulator, and has an inhibiting effect on certain inflammatory markers.[12] Various animal and human studies support the use of curcumin in promoting health in joints, gastrointestinal mucosa, and neural cells, and in protecting against and destroying amyloid plaques in the brain. An article titled "Protective Effects of Indian Spice Curcumin Against Amyloid Beta in Alzheimer's Disease" published by the National Institutes of Health (NIH) in February 2018 said, "Recent research on amyloid-β and curcumin has revealed that curcumin prevents amyloid-β aggregation and crosses the blood brain barrier (BBB), reaches brain cells and protects neurons from various toxic insults of aging and amyloid-β in humans."[13] The typical dose in human studies ranges from 3.75 mg to 1,200 mg per day.

Blueberries

Blueberries are rich in the antioxidants known as *anthocyanins*. In a study with nine elderly human participants, a team at the University of Cincinnati found that compared to a comparable group that was given a placebo, participants who were given blueberry juice scored higher on memory tests, had improved word list recall, and experienced fewer depressive symptoms.[14] Berries of all types—strawberries, raspberries, and blackberries—bring you critical minerals, vitamins, antioxidants, flavonoids, polyphenols, and a host of other important phytonutrients that are good for your brain and your heart.

Greens

Ideally, according to the Institute of Functional Medicine, we should eat five to nine servings of greens a day. Both one cup of raw greens and half a cup of cooked vegetables count as servings. The best greens to eat are the dark leafy ones like spinach and kale, as well as cruciferous vegetables. Broccoli, cauliflower, cabbage, brussels sprouts, and collard greens are all cruciferous vegetables. These vegetables affect the way the liver detoxifies chemicals, thereby supporting the detoxification system. Cruciferous vegetables can be harder to digest, so lightly steaming them for five minutes at less than 118 degrees can help the mineral content become more bioavailable without overcooking the vegetable and destroying its vitamins.

In 2015, researchers at Rush University in Chicago evaluated the diet and mental function of 950 elderly people. After adjusting for variables such as education, exercise, and family history of dementia, the researchers found that those participants who ate leafy green vegetables such as spinach and kale once or twice a day experienced significantly less cognitive decline than those who didn't. In fact, participants who ate greens halted their mental decline by an average of eleven years.[15]

Legumes

Legumes such as peas, beans, and lentils are health superfoods loaded with fiber. Not only are they inexpensive, they are also apparently very good for our health and longevity.

Ocean Robbins of the Food Revolution Network stated the following in 2018: "In 2004, researchers from Japan, Sweden, Greece, and Australia teamed up for a fascinating study. They wanted to see if there was any one food group that was consistently linked with a longer lifespan in every nation and group. And they found one: legumes. Whether it was the Swedes dining on brown beans and peas, the Japanese eating soy, or the people living around the Mediterranean and enjoying chickpeas, lentils, and white beans, one thing was clear: the more legumes people ate, the longer they lived. As the researchers looked at data across all the populations combined, legumes were the food that showed up with the most plausible, consistent, and statistically significant results. Over the course of the study, every 20-g (2-tbsp.) increase in daily legume consumption was correlated with an 8 percent reduction in the risk of death."[16]

The legume family includes thousands of colorful varieties of beans, peas, lentils, soybeans, and even peanuts. They grow in pods, and like nuts and seeds, each legume has the potential to sprout and grow into a new plant. Try to have 2 tbsp., or 20 g, a day.

Coffee

Coffee has been somewhat controversial. Shared by billions of people worldwide, it's been thought of as overly stimulating, acidifying, exacerbating fatigue by masking it, and continuing to add adrenalin to a system that should instead be resting. Fortunately, there's also a lot of evidence that coffee brings some significant benefits. Coffee is a vasodilator, opening the blood vessels and improving circulation.

Ocean Robbins of the Food Revolution Network writes this:

> *The Cardiovascular Risk Factors, Aging and Dementia study tracked more than 1,500 randomly selected Finnish people for 21 years, examining a broad range of diet and lifestyle choices and how they correlated with health outcomes. The study found that when people at midlife drank 3–5 cups of coffee per day (which sounds like a lot!), they had as they grew older, compared to non-coffee drinkers, a 65% decreased risk of dementia. A 13-year study of more than 80,000 Japanese adults found those who drank at least one cup of coffee per day had a 20% reduced risk of stroke.*[17]

And in another study, 34,670 women in Sweden were tracked for more than ten years. Those who did not drink any coffee were at elevated risk of stroke, while the women who drank at least one cup per day reduced their risk of stroke by 22 to 25 percent.[18]

Coffee consumption has also been shown to be good for your reaction time, memory, vigilance, and general cognitive function. If you tend to be an anxious person, then I would avoid coffee and stick with tea instead.

Tea

The story of tea began in China. Tea became the national drink of China around 700 CE, although it was discovered by a Chinese emperor, Shen Nung, in 2737 BCE, when some leaves from a tree dropped into a pot of boiling water that he drank by accident. There are four types of tea: white, green, oolong, and black. White and green tea are the least processed and have the most antioxidants and the lowest levels of caffeine.

Tea consumption has been linked to reduced rates of Alzheimer's disease.[19]

Tea does contain caffeine, but at about a third the rate of coffee per cup. If you steep your tea bag for sixty seconds, dump out the water, and then re-steep it, you are essentially brewing a cup of decaffeinated tea. This will be better for you if you tend toward anxiety with caffeine. Try it plain, with milk and honey, or with a squeeze of lemon.

Vitamins and Minerals

My patients sometimes ask me a very good question: "Is it really necessary to supplement with extra vitamins and minerals?"

The short answer is "No, as long as you are eating wild, fresh, whole, organic, local, non-genetically modified foods grown in virgin mineral and nutrient-rich soils, freshly picked and not transported across vast distances or stored for months." Since most of us live busy lives, eat out more than we cook at home, don't grow vegetables in our backyard garden, and don't have the ability to source all our foods from optimal sources such as local farmers' markets, I recommend an intelligent approach to supplementing your diet with certain high-quality vitamins and minerals.

Vitamins act as cofactors that run all aspects of our biochemistry. If our vitamin intake is insufficient, serious illness can occur. Most of us are not getting enough vitamins and minerals. I find that inevitably my patients feel better, their energy improves, and their mental clarity and resilience are enhanced when they take a good multivitamin and mineral complex containing at least the following:

- B-complex
- Lithium
- Magnesium
- Omega-3 fats (already discussed)
- Phytonutrient-rich multivitamins (see information further down under the Basic Plan)
- Selenium
- Vitamin D
- Zinc

Let's take a closer look at these essential vitamins and minerals.

B Complex

The B vitamins, specifically 1, 2, 3, 6, 9, and 12, play an important role in brain health. They boost the production of neurotransmitters, those chemicals that deliver messages via the neurons between the brain and body. Our bodies don't store B vitamins, so we need to eat them or take a supplement of them daily in our foods. Foods that have B vitamins are whole grains, red meat, poultry, fish, eggs, milk, cheese, legumes, seeds, nuts, and dark leafy vegetables. The most crucial B vitamins are B6, B9 (also called folic acid), and B12. These three types of B vitamins provide help with a biochemical process in your body called *methylation*, which helps your entire body's biochemistry. B12 vitamin is crucial for the normal functioning of the brain and the nervous system. It is also involved in the formation of red blood cells and helps to create and regulate DNA. The metabolism of every cell in the body depends on vitamin B12, as it plays a part in the synthesis of fatty acids and energy production. We source B12 and other B vitamins from meat, red meat in particular. For vegetarians who do not eat meat, this is a very important vitamin to supplement with.

Lithium

The World Health Organization lists lithium as one of the nutritionally essential trace elements, alongside zinc, iodine, and others. Most of us get our lithium from tap water. Lithium is not only good for emotional mood issues but is also able to curb Alzheimer's dementia. Lithium's effectiveness in suicide prevention has also been demonstrated. Substantial medical literature also exists to support the use of lithium in a broad spectrum of other neurological conditions, including substance abuse, violent and aggressive behavior, ADHD, and cognitive decline. Lithium has been shown to influence the expression of over fifty different genes. Working in these epigenetic pathways, lithium supports a wide range of neuroprotective and neurotrophic actions that literally change brain plasticity.

Lithium has been shown to disrupt a key enzyme responsible for the development of the undesirable amyloid plaques and neurofibrillary tangles associated with Alzheimer's, which are caused by increased activity of the enzyme glycogen synthase kinase 3β (GSK3B). Lithium works as a direct GSK3B inhibitor, halting inappropriate amyloid production. Lithium ions also help the brain repair from damage that has already happened in Alzheimer's, by encouraging the synthesis and release of key neurotrophic factors such as brain derived nerve growth factor (BDNF) and neurotrophin-3 (NT-3), which stimulate the growth and repair of neurons.

People taking lithium have been found to have significantly higher gray matter volume. Nerve cells exposed to lithium respond by increasing in dendritic number and length. This is from an article titled "Lithium Treatment Increases Gray Matter Volume in Human Brain, WSU Researchers Find" from Oct 6, 2000:

> *Dr. Gregory Moore, director of Brain Imaging Research Center at Wayne State University's School of Medicine, led a study to see whether or not lithium could increase the brain's gray matter, the part of the brain that is most involved with memory and thinking. Shockingly after 4 weeks of taking lithium … study participants had significantly increased their brain's gray matter.*

So how much lithium should we take? It's safe to take 20 mg of lithium orotate without guidance. In the body, minerals come as a balance, so it is best to measure your mineral levels. This can be done by testing blood, urine, or hair during an appointment at my office. To locate my offices in order to book an appointment, go my website: www.drjacqueline.com.

Fortunately, for the first time in human history we live in an age when scientists are beginning to understand that by optimizing micronutrients and making a few simple lifestyle changes, our brains can be healthy and we can continue to be sharp into our old age!

Magnesium

Magnesium is one of the most essential minerals. It is involved in over three hundred enzyme processes and is needed to generate adenosine triphosphate (ATP), our body's source of energy. Magnesium is so important that it's used in emergency rooms when a person is dying of a life-threatening arrhythmia. Amazingly, up to half of all Americans are deficient in magnesium without knowing it. For example, magnesium is involved in the formation of nucleic proteins in the body, in cell growth and division, and in the electrolyte composition in our cells. It is necessary for the vasomotor tone of our blood vessels, neuromusculoskeletal contraction, and vitamin D metabolism, and it is essential for our sleep.

In an article posted by Sayer Ji of GreenMedInfo on October 3, 2019, Ali Le Vere, BS, wrote this:

> *Food processing and industrial agriculture, including monoculture crop practices and the use of magnesium-devoid fertilizers, have led to soil erosion and depletion of magnesium content in our food. Magnesium is likewise removed from most drinking water supplies, rendering magnesium deficiency an inevitability. As such, our daily intake of magnesium has steadily declined from 500 milligrams (mg) per day to 175 mg per day. The nutrient-poor, energy-dense dietary patterns which have come to dominate the industrialized landscape are also insufficient in the fiber-rich fruits and vegetables which contain magnesium.*

Magnesium acts as an antidepressant through specific biological systems. Magnesium operates as an agonist, or a stimulatory molecule, for γ-aminobutyric acid (GABA) receptors. GABA is the main inhibitory neurotransmitter in the central nervous system. By binding to the GABA receptor and replicating the effects of GABA, magnesium may alleviate anxiety. Magnesium may also elicit its antidepressant effects by acting as an inorganic antagonist of N-methyl-d-aspartic acid (NMDA) receptor function. Receptor antagonists are ligands, or substances which bind to a receptor but inhibit its activity rather than activating it. NMDA receptors, which occur on the surface of nerve cells, are activated in part by glutamate, one of the excitatory amino acids in the brain.

Researchers state that dysfunction of NMDA receptors seems to play a crucial role in the neurobiology of disorders such as Parkinson's disease, Alzheimer's disease, epilepsy, ischemic stroke, anxiety, and depression, such that ligands interacting with different sites of NMDA receptor complex are widely investigated as potential agents for the treatment of a variety of neuropsychiatric disorders.[20] In fact, drug inhibitors at the NMDA receptor complex, such as ketamine, demonstrate antidepressant effects but also induce such severe side effects that their clinical utility is limited. Magnesium, on the other hand, may have a similar mechanism of action by interfering with NMDA receptor activation without the adverse consequences of drug-induced NMDA receptor blockade.

Let me highlight a few studies here:

- In a randomized trial of elderly patients with **type 2 diabetes** and magnesium deficiency, elemental magnesium administered at 450 mg per day was found to have equivalent efficacy to 50 mg of the antidepressant drug Imipramine in treating depressive symptoms.
- Magnesium citrate taken at 300 mg per day has likewise been shown to decrease depression and other symptoms in patients with fibromyalgia as indicated by significant decreases in the **fibromyalgia** impact questionnaire (FIQ) and Beck depression scores.
- A recent open-label, randomized, cross-over trial was conducted in outpatient primary care clinics on 126 adults diagnosed with depression. During the intervention, 248 mg of elemental magnesium chloride per day, obtained from four 500 mg tablets, was administered for six weeks and compared to six weeks of no treatment, and subjects were evaluated for changes in depressive symptoms. Magnesium administration results in clinically significant improvements in scores on both the Patient Health Questionnaire-9, a validated measure of the severity of depression and response to treatment, and the Generalized Anxiety Disorders-7 (GAD-7), a sensitive self-reported screening tool for severity of anxiety disorders. Impressively, results appeared in as little as two weeks, representing the dramatic improvement that nutrient restoration can facilitate. Magnesium exerted antidepressant effects regardless of baseline magnesium levels. It also exhibited efficacy independent of the gender, age, or baseline

> severity of depression of subjects, as well as their use of antidepressant medications. The authors of the study conclude, "Magnesium is effective for mild-to-moderate depression in adults. It works quickly and is well tolerated without the need for close monitoring for toxicity."[21]

Researchers note that "low magnesium intakes and blood levels have been associated with type 2 diabetes, metabolic syndrome, elevated C-reactive protein, hypertension, atherosclerotic vascular disease, sudden cardiac death, osteoporosis, migraine headache, asthma, and colon cancer." In addition, magnesium deficiency at a cellular level "elicits calcium-activated inflammatory cascades independent of injury or pathogens." Low magnesium is associated with systemic inflammation, and inflammation is at the root of most chronic and degenerative diseases.[22]

The Problem with Magnesium Level Testing

While the first inclination of some physicians may be to test magnesium levels for an objective parameter of deficiency, the widely used serum, or plasma, magnesium test does not accurately reflect magnesium levels stored in other tissues. In addition, both this hematological index of magnesium status, referred to as *total magnesium*, and the erythrocyte magnesium level, indicative of the levels of magnesium inside red blood cells, are not negatively affected until severe magnesium deprivation has occurred. Therefore, these testing methodologies are not accurate enough to catch preliminary or subclinical magnesium deficiency. My choice for testing magnesium levels is either as red blood cell (RBC) elements or through hair analysis, which I cover in the "Lab Work" section.

Good food sources of magnesium include pumpkin and squash seed kernels, Brazil nuts, almonds, cashews, peanuts, pine nuts, quinoa, spinach, Swiss chard, beet greens, potatoes, artichoke hearts, dates, bananas, coconut milk, prickly pears, black beans, lima beans, soybeans, and seafood, including halibut, abalone, anchovies, caviar, conch, crabs, oysters, scallops, snails, and pollock. However, it is important to note that magnesium can leach from vegetables when food is boiled, and that too much fiber can decrease magnesium absorption by increasing gastrointestinal motility.

Which Type of Magnesium Supplement Should I Take?

Organic salts of magnesium—including the acetate, ascorbate, aspartate, bicitrate, gluconate, and lactate forms—are more soluble and biologically active than magnesium mineral salts such as magnesium oxide, magnesium carbonate, magnesium chloride, and magnesium sulfate.

However, case studies have shown remarkably rapid recovery from major depression, in less than seven days, when magnesium glycinate and magnesium taurinate are administered at dosages of 125–300 mg with each meal and at bedtime. Magnesium threonate may also be explored as a therapeutic option, as it may have better penetration through the blood-brain barrier to restore neurological levels of magnesium. This form, which is delivered directly to the brain, may improve cerebral signaling pathways and synaptic connections between nerve cells, as well as support learning and memory, although the studies have only been conducted in animal models.

Researchers report that magnesium is usually effective for treating depression in general use, and that comorbid conditions occurring in these case studies, including "traumatic brain injury, headache, suicidal ideation, anxiety, irritability, insomnia, postpartum depression, cocaine, alcohol and tobacco abuse, hypersensitivity to calcium, short-term memory loss and IQ loss were also benefited" by magnesium supplementation.[23]

The Institute of Medicine sets the upper tolerable limit for intake, barring abnormal kidney function, at 350 mg of elemental magnesium per day, but there are few adverse side effects documented, unless consumed in inordinate doses.

Before changing your medication or nutraceutical regimen, always consult a functional or integrative medical doctor for contraindications. However, given the benign nature of magnesium supplementation and the ubiquity of magnesium insufficiency, those who are depressed should consider this as a first-line strategy.

This quote is from an article by the American Osteopathic Association, published in *Science Daily* on February 26, 2018:

> *Up to 50 percent of the US population is magnesium deficient. Vitamin D can't be metabolized without sufficient magnesium levels, meaning vitamin D remains stored and inactive for as many as 50 percent of Americans.*

Standard serum, or blood, levels of magnesium do not accurately reflect body magnesium levels. The best way to know if you have enough magnesium is through red blood cell content of magnesium or a blood test based on white blood cell growth in a medium with magnesium. I like to use a lab called Spectracell for all micronutrient testing. Think of magnesium as the relaxation mineral. If there is stiffness or cramping in your body or brain, you may need more of it. Conditions such as an anxious, "tight" mood; a head "tight" with headaches; or bowels "tight" from constipation are most likely due to magnesium deficiency. Magnesium inhibits platelet aggregation, dilates blood vessels, and acts as an antispasmodic on muscles. Unfortunately, very few doctors actually prescribe magnesium supplementation. If you seek optimal brain performance, you will need magnesium. Many reputable research studies show magnesium to be helpful with heart attacks, asthma, migraines, premenstrual syndrome, pregnancy issues, urinary problems, diabetes, hypoglycemia, hypertension, sickle-cell disease, and even alcohol withdrawal.

The dosage I recommend is based on the studies quoted previously: 125–300 mg magnesium glycinate or taurinate once or up to three times a day with meals. You can start with a once-a-day dose, and if you don't feel much better, increase this dose. If you begin to have loose stools, then you likely have too much magnesium in your system and you can back down.

Phytonutrients

Phytonutrients are the nutritional components of our vegetables and fruits that make them brightly colored, such as the red in raspberries, the purple in grapes, and the orange in sweet potatoes. I prescribe a multivitamin that has phytonutrients in it and has scientifically demonstrated phytonutrient potential for antioxidant protection to defend cellular health and DNA stability, verified by sophisticated in vitro ORACFN and Comet assays. The following is a list of phytonutrients in the multivitamin PhytoMulti:

- 400 mg Citrus bioflavonoid complex
- Green coffee bean extract
- Pomegranate whole fruit extract
- Grape seed extract
- Blueberry (Vaccinium spp.) fruit extract
- Green tea leaf extract
- Bitter melon fruit extract
- Prune skin extract
- Watercress aerial parts
- Chinese cinnamon (*Cinnamomum cassia*) bark powder
- Indian gum arabic tree bark and heartwood extract
- Rosemary extract
- Artichoke leaf extract

Read more about PhytoMulti in this PDF.

Selenium

Selenium is a powerful antioxidant that is critical for brain health. Selenium is a cofactor for glutathione peroxidase, the most important antioxidant for the brain and liver, and is known to be about one thousand times more potent as an antioxidant than vitamins E and C. Selenium also has antiviral effects and enhances the immune system. Animal studies have shown it to help prevent cancer and viral illnesses. According to WebMD, a reputable source of health information, the amount of selenium in soil varies a lot around the world, which means that the foods grown in these soils also have differing selenium levels. In the US, the Eastern Coastal Plain and the Pacific Northwest have the lowest selenium levels. People in these regions naturally take in about 60 to 90 mcg of selenium per day from their diet. Although this amount of selenium is adequate, it is below the average daily intake in the US, which is 125 mcg.

> *Selenium is used for [combatting] diseases of the heart and blood vessels, including stroke and "hardening of the arteries" (atherosclerosis). It is also used for preventing various cancers, including cancer of the prostate, stomach, lung, and skin.*[24]

Vitamin D

It's hard to decide which one vitamin is the most important, but vitamin D certainly ranks among the top contenders. We need vitamin D for so many things, including production of serotonin (our "happy mood" neurotransmitter), activating our thyroid hormone, shuttling amyloid protein out of the brain, and aiding our immune system in determining which immune T helper cells to activate. Vitamin D is first captured when we expose our bare skin to direct sunlight. After sunlight contacts our skin, it gets converted into a biologically active form by our kidneys. Sunblock with a sun protection factor (SPF) higher than 14 will block vitamin D from getting into your skin from the sun.

Unfortunately, deficiency in vitamin D affects over a third of the population. The *British Journal of Nutrition* recently reported this:

> *Vitamin D deficiency (VDD) and insufficiency (VDI) are increasing at a global level, and they are associated with increased risk of various diseases. Serum 25-hydroxyvitamin D 25(OH) measurements were*

collected from 26,010 adults aged ≥18 years from the National Health and Nutrition Examination Survey (NHANES) 2001-2010. Using thresholds recommended by the Endocrine Society, vitamin D deficiency was defined as 25(OH)D<50 nmol/L. The prevalence of vitamin D deficiency in 2001-2010 was 28·9%.[25]

Vitamin D deficiency is frequently undiagnosed, even though it has been linked to depression, dementia, fibromyalgia, high blood pressure, diabetes, muscle pain, bone loss, and autoimmune diseases such as multiple sclerosis. Since we tend to use sunblock on our skin for fear of getting skin cancer, most of us aren't getting enough exposure to sunlight. Nevertheless, we need to expose our skin for fifteen minutes uninterrupted in the noonday sun—with no skin protection on—in order to absorb a sufficient amount. Few people can get outside for that long in the sun. Over the years, I have tested my patients' vitamin D levels, and almost everyone tests low, so to be safe I recommend vitamin D supplements to ensure adequate amounts. Be careful not to be overzealous with vitamin D supplementation, however, as one can become toxic in vitamin D. It takes a lot to get toxic, over 100 international units (IU) in the blood, which would mean taking 10,000 IU a day for months. If you are taking vitamin D on a regular basis, please have your blood level checked after a couple of months. Vitamin D has many beneficial effects for the brain. It's needed to make the important neurotransmitter serotonin, which allows us to feel calm and happy and to sleep well.

According to a 2019 article in *Experimental Neurobiology*,

Vitamin D levels in rats have been shown to help the blood-brain barrier.[26]

A more recent discovery about vitamin D is that it can usher out the amyloid protein from the brain. Amyloid protein is found in Alzheimer's dementia, creating tangles in the brain. Many of the pharmaceutical trials have aimed at lowering amyloid protein production in the brain, with the hopes that Alzheimer's dementia can be avoided. Most of these medications have failed. However, simply optimizing our vitamin D levels can help in this regard through a specific receptor called *lipoprotein receptor-related protein* (LRP-1). LRP-1 has also been identified as an amyloid beta scavenger receptor that can remove amyloid beta from the brain through the blood-brain barrier. However, its expression is decreased in people with neurological dysfunction. A review points to recent evidence that after supplementation with *the active form of vitamin D, 1,25-(OH)2D3*, LRP-1 expression increases significantly both in vivo and in vitro. This is because so many vitamin D receptors are expressed in the brain.[27]

Several studies also suggest that deficiency, or inhibition, in the receptor to which vitamin D binds in the body (vitamin D receptor, or VDR) could be a risk factor for neurodegenerative disease. The presence of this VDR-receptor defect can be detected in a blood lab test for genetic pathway defects.

During my own process of healing my brain, I discovered that I had low serotonin production and a genetic abnormality in my vitamin D receptor site. I have supplemented with extra vitamin D and the herb St. John's Wort for several years now and have found a solid emotional resiliency within. I used to feel low and be tearful very easily. Now, I feel like I have a solid core within and a sense of fulfillment at all times.

Zinc

More than a third of the world's population is zinc deficient, which is alarming because zinc is used by enzymes in the body more than any other mineral. Zinc helps heal wounds, enhances immune function, reduces inflammation, has direct and indirect antiviral effects, and promotes the conversion of inactive thyroid to active thyroid. Double-blind clinical trials have shown zinc to also be beneficial for acne, colds, rheumatoid arthritis, psoriatic arthritis, gastric ulcers, macular degeneration, growth retardation, anorexia nervosa, and tinnitus. Low levels of zinc have been linked to ADHD, autism, depression, and even schizophrenia.

The Basic Plan to Optimize Nutrition for Brain Health

In light of all I have said above, here are the key components of my nutrition plan for brain health.

Eat More Vegetables, Fruits, and Non-farmed Fish

In summary, these fifteen dietary components have been shown to powerfully impact neurological function:

Beans and legumes

Berries

Coffee

Colored vegetables

Grass-fed meats (limited to four servings a week)

Green leafy vegetables

Healthy oils (olive oil, coconut oil, avocado oil, sesame oil)

Nuts (almonds, macadamia, walnuts, pecans)

Omega-3 eggs

Poultry (organic pasture-raised)

Seeds (pumpkin, flaxseeds, hempseeds, chia)

Tea

Turmeric spice

Wild fatty fish

Wine (limited amounts, ranging from two glasses a week to one glass a day)

Avoid or Reduce These Brain-Damaging Foods

While filling up with healthy nutrients is optimal, you also need to reduce other foods that impair the natural functioning of the brain.

Butter or margarine to under one tbsp. per day

Cheese to under one serving a week

Eliminate all toxic fats (trans fats, soy, canola oil, safflower oil)

Fried or fast foods to under one serving a week

Gluten

Pastries and sweets to under two servings a week

Processed foods with food coloring or highly modified GMO crops such as corn, soy, and vegetable oils

Red meat to under four servings a week

Optimize Nutrition with Supplements

I recommend my patients take a full-spectrum multivitamin and mineral daily. I carry my favorite brand, Metagenics Phytonutrients, which you can learn about here and purchase at the end of the book in the resources section.

B-complex, 25–100 mg a day

Lithium, 20–40 mg a day

Magnesium, 200–300 mg once or twice a day

Omega-3 fats, 2,000–4,000 mg a day

Selenium, 200 mcg a day

Vitamin D3, 5,000–10,000 IU a day

Zinc, 25 mg a day

Fasting

Fast twelve to sixteen hours between dinner and breakfast or do a whole-day fast once a week. According to a study published in the February 2017 issue of *Aging Cell*, tests in Brazil showed that fasting increases the amount of calcium the mitochondria in neurons can hold onto.[28] By collecting extra calcium, the mitochondria can protect neurons from being damaged by what's called *excitotoxicity*—a destructive reaction to the neurotransmitter glutamate. When a neuron overreacts to glutamate, the reaction resembles what happens to your TV set when lightning hits your house. A lightning voltage surge can cause TV circuits to be overloaded and fried, destroying your TV set. In the brain, excitotoxicity does something like that—overwhelming and burning up neurons. Extra calcium in mitochondria, which is what happens when we fast, is like a surge protector that keeps the overload from putting neurons out of commission. An additional benefit to intermittent fasting is that it makes mitochondria more adaptable in how they react to available nutrients in the cell—switching from processing sugars to fats. Tests show fasting helps mitochondria metabolize fat more effectively.[29]

Of course, all of these benefits don't happen just in brain cells. They're widespread in the body. That's a key reason why researchers keep doing detailed tests on fasting and exercise. Together they're becoming the dynamic duo of preventive medicine. All-out fasting is a challenge for most of us, which is why intermittent fasting has become so popular. The easiest approach is to make sure that at least twelve hours pass between your last meal of the day and your first meal in the morning. Much more effective is to wait sixteen hours between the first and last meals—meaning you do all your eating during an eight-hour window—perhaps from 10:00 a.m. to 6:00 p.m.[30]

Lab Work

Depending upon your individual circumstances, it may be important to supplement the lifestyle aspects of good brain nutrition with specific laboratory tests. Your doctor can test for deficiencies in amino acids and neurotransmitters through urine or blood collection. If you are really low in amino acids and your body is not absorbing them from your food because your gut health is compromised (see chapter 5, "Healing Leaky Gut and Healing Leaky Brain"), your doctor may arrange for you to receive intravenous (IV) nutrient therapy. This can rapidly affect and improve your overall health and nutrition.

Blood tests can be done for the following key nutrients: omega-3 fats, vitamin D, magnesium, selenium, zinc, B12, and coenzyme Q10 (CoQ10), as well as for vitamin D receptor-site genetic abnormalities. The results of your lab testing can get you on a solid supplement and dietary regime to help maximize the building blocks you need for your brain health. Sometimes simply improving one's nutrition, both through whole foods and supplements, can make one feel better in a matter of weeks! Unfortunately, most hospital-based or standard laboratories do not offer blood testing for all of the above nutrients; recall also that magnesium plasma levels are often inaccurate. I use a lab called Doctor's Data, and on some occasions I do hair testing if a blood lab is not available in the patient's geographic area. Doctor's Data has been validated since 1972 as a supplier of trace-element results for the certification of hair reference material to the European Commission's Joint Research Centre. Hair is essentially an excretory tissue and will reflect low mineral levels if they have been dropping in a person's diet for several months. Hair will also show toxic elements such as mercury or arsenic (covered in chapter 6). The hair follicle contains protein that incorporates elements permanently into the hair with no further exchange or equilibration with other tissues. Nutrient elements, including magnesium, chromium, zinc, copper, and selenium, are obligatory cofactors for hundreds of important enzymes and also are essential for the normal functions of vitamins. The level of these elements in hair correlates with levels in organs and other tissues. Scalp hair is easy to sample because it grows an average of 1–2 cm per month and contains a "temporal record" of element metabolism and exposure to toxic elements.

Interrelationship of Hormones and Minerals

In this chapter we have focused on the importance of minerals. It turns out minerals and hormones have an important interrelationship regarding our brain health. For example, our hormones need zinc, selenium, manganese, magnesium, and vitamin A in order to be produced in the right amounts. When our hormones are adequately supplied with such minerals, they are able to function properly, allowing for optimal communication and regulatory activity. If minerals are not in adequate supply—or if there are other limiting factors affecting the levels of our hormones—we can experience fatigue, depression, anxiety, memory problems, weight gain, and a sluggish immune system. The symphony of the body goes out of tune and the subtle melody of good health is not produced.

It is important to bear in mind, however, that hormone production drops naturally with age. For example, by age thirty-five, dehydroepiandrosterone (DHEA) production goes down by 20 percent. Stress also causes hormone production to drop. But we can combat that decline in hormone production with improved diet and by supplementing with exogenous DHEA and other hormones under the guidance of a physician.

4 | BALANCING HEALTHY HORMONES

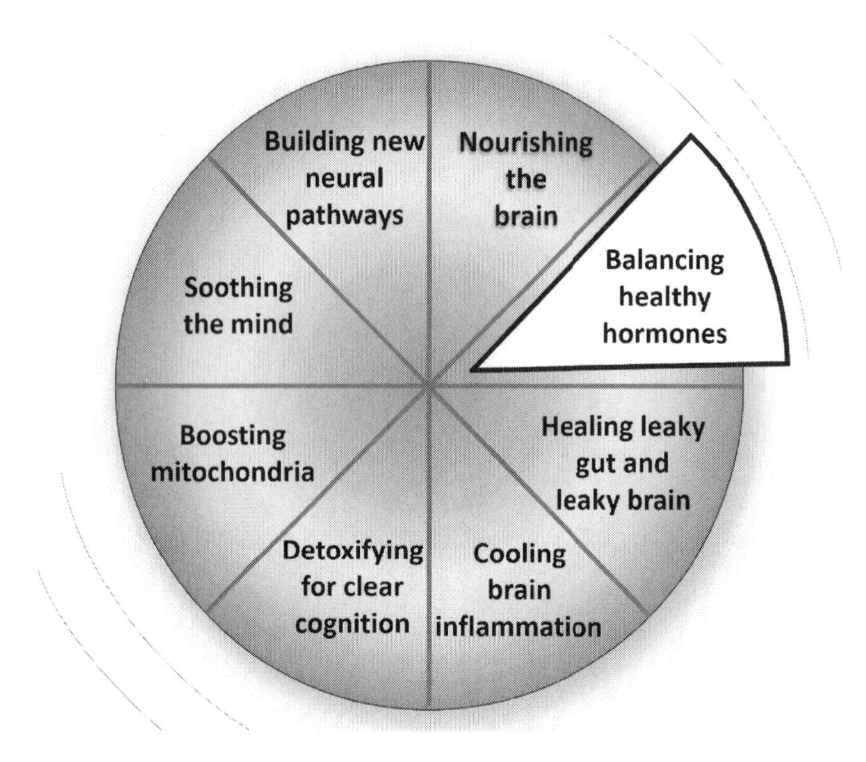

Hormones are a special class of biomolecules that are produced within our endocrine organs. They are designed to carry messages to our cells to regulate the production of other important molecules in the body. Think of your hormones as being on-off switches that the body uses to regulate levels of a wide spectrum of important molecules needed for optimal health. Hormones produce effects throughout the whole body in a finely orchestrated symphony and are part of a larger communication system in our bodies.

Major categories of hormones include the following groups:

Adrenal hormones—this group of hormones give us immediate energy: cortisol, epinephrine, norepinephrine, pregnenolone, and DHEA; these hormones are produced by the adrenal glands, which sit on top of the kidneys.

Insulin—this allows for healthy glucose metabolism to operate within each of our cells and is made by the pancreas.

Melatonin—produced by the pineal gland, this helps us to sleep and regenerate our brain.

Metabolic hormone or thyroid hormone—this is produced by the thyroid gland, the endocrine gland which optimizes our body's use of oxygen.

Neurotransmitters—these are the biochemical messengers of the nervous system such as serotonin, dopamine, acetylcholine, and gamma-aminobutyric acid (GABA). We have fifty in total, but the ones I mention in this book are the most common.

Sex hormones—these help with mucous-membrane health, bone strength, focus, drive, libido, and memory: estrogen, progesterone, and testosterone (from your ovaries, adrenals, or testes).

Each of these hormones is produced by certain glands in the body. Three very important endocrine glands are located in the brain: the pituitary, the hypothalamus, and the pineal gland. Since these hormones are helping the exquisite balance in your body, these balancing acts can be thought of in the following ways:

Blood sugar balance—this is modulated by insulin produced by your pancreas, which lies deep underneath most of your intestines just to the left of your spine in your abdomen.

Growth, sleep, and mood—this is balanced through the pineal gland in the deep middle and back of the brain, as well as through the adrenals, sex organs, pituitary gland, and hypothalamus. As an example, let's look at the pituitary gland—a master endocrine organ in the brain that is located just behind the eyes. The pituitary gland releases thyroid stimulating hormone (TSH), which stimulates the thyroid gland to make the thyroid hormones thyroxine (T3), levothyroxine (T4), follicle stimulating hormone (FSH), and luteinizing hormone (LH) (FSH stimulates the ovaries in a woman and LH stimulates the testicles in a man), and adrenocorticotropic releasing hormone (ACTH), which stimulates the adrenal gland. Our hormones help us modulate and adapt to the circumstances in our day, as well as the pressures in our life. They help us remain resilient and support our function as we get older. They are necessary for the regeneration of our brain and nervous system.

Metabolism—this is regulated through your thyroid gland.

Sexual behavior and function—this is regulated through the hypothalamus, pituitary gland, and genital organs, being ovaries if you are a woman or testes if you are a man.

The stress response—this is modulated by your pituitary gland and hypothalamus in your brain and through your adrenal glands, which sit right on top of your kidneys.

Neurotransmitters and Brain Function

Our body makes essential chemicals called neurotransmitters, which are fundamental in almost every function in our body. Each nerve cell releases different types of neurotransmitters, which seek out receptors on other cells, bind to them, and communicate instructions. As far as our brain's health is concerned, neurotransmitters are key players in mood regulation and memory. Neurotransmission is how the brain cells communicate with one another, by producing chemicals that travel in between the synapses of the nerve cells. Neurotransmission can be affected by the quantity and quality of the neurotransmitters produced and by how well these molecules bind to their receptors. When our neurotransmission is "off," we may have symptoms like these:

Being more distracted

Having difficulty remembering names of places or people and relying on phrases such as "you know what I mean" when trying to cover up poor recall

Losing our train of thought

Taking longer to retrieve memories

Thinking that we are listening but realizing we don't remember what the person just said

The neurotransmitters that are critical for brain function are these:

Acetylcholine is in charge of supporting our memory.

Dopamine is responsible for attention, focus, pleasure, and reward.

GABA is a neurotransmitter that calms the brain.

Serotonin is the "happy" molecule; lack of it leads to depression.

These brain neurotransmitters work together. Dopamine and acetylcholine excite and stimulate you, whereas serotonin and GABA relax you and calm you down. When you have a good balance of these excitatory and inhibitory neurotransmitters flowing through your system, you will feel aware, calm, and quietly joyous. Psychiatric medicines—such as Prozac, Paxil, Zoloft, Effexor, Cymbalta, and Wellbutrin to name a few—increase the presence of neurotransmitters by inhibiting their breakdown. But these medicines don't address the question of *why* our neurotransmitters are low in the first place!

The factors interfering with our brain's biochemistry—and thus adversely affecting our neurotransmitters—include the following:

- Amino acid deficiency in the diet (especially true for vegetarians)
- Genetic disorders that affect brain chemistry (such as the MTHFR gene SNP)
- High levels of stress
- Inflammation of the brain (from trauma, autoimmune conditions, or stress)
- Leaky gut-brain axis
- Specific nutrient deficiencies (such as vitamin D or omega-3s)
- Toxins such as heavy metals that interfere with the binding of neurotransmitters to receptor sites. We can get heavy metal exposure from dental amalgams, eating a lot of tuna fish, or tap water from old leaded pipes (covered in chapter 7).

Let me tell you a story about a forty-nine-year-old professor of psychology who came to me with irregular periods, hip pain, and emotional stress from the pressure of writing her third book. She was married and had a teenage son. At the time, her irregular periods weren't causing any hot flashes or serious side effects, but her husband did think she was moodier than usual. She was drinking one espresso in the morning and getting chiropractic care and massage therapy. She ate well and took multivitamins, fish oil, and an amino acid called DL-phenylalanine for her mood, yet she still felt anxious.

After her initial visit with me, I ordered a panel of urine, blood, and saliva tests to look at her hormones. I put her on a key supplement to increase her dopamine production and thereby support her motivation and focus with her book. Upon her three-month follow-up, she said she had a "huge revelation" with the supplement I gave her to raise her dopamine. She said she had significantly more energy and clarity and that her mood was great. The anxiety which she used to experience upon waking each morning had disappeared. We reviewed her labs at that time, and I noticed that her levels of cortisol (a key hormone produced by the adrenal glands) were about a third of normal. I began her on a low dose of cortisol and an estrogen patch containing a plant-based hormone. After another three months, she returned to me saying, "I feel so much better I don't even know how to describe it. I've never felt this good in my life!"

At our original visit she had said her energy was a "2 out of 10," and after approximately six months she described her energy as "10 out of 10." To top it off, she had finished her manuscript with time to spare! Prior to the cortisol prescription she was crying in her husband's lap and thinking she couldn't make it. Her writing became easy.

The following hormones help control our energy, focus, mood, and memory:

DHEA
Cortisol
Estrogen
Pregnenolone
Progesterone
Testosterone
Thyroid

Sex Hormones

Our sex hormones do more than just regulate our libido and fertility. Women's sex hormones—estrogen, progesterone, and testosterone—are produced by the ovaries and later in life by the adrenals. Let's look at each one.

Estrogen

Estrogen makes you feel sensual, bringing a glow to your skin, moisture to your eyes, fullness to your breasts, clarity to your mind, lubrication to your vagina, and an overall sense of womanness.

In the article "Cognition and Memory" that appeared in the January 2013 issue of *Women's International Pharmacy*, it was reported that "estrogen promotes networking between brain cells by increasing the number of dendritic branches and keeping them strong and well-defined, which also increases the number of potential synapses."

Estrogen increases levels of mood-regulating neurotransmitters such as acetylcholine, serotonin, and noradrenaline. It also increases the density of neurotransmitter receptors. Finally, estrogen maintains the health of the nerve cell by encouraging nerve growth and preventing the accumulation of free radicals, reducing inflammation, and promoting increased blood flow. Dr. Dale Bredesen observed in his studies on Alzheimer's disease that there was an increased risk for dementia when hormones such as estrogen drop in postmenopausal women. Dr. Barbara Sherwin, professor emerita at McGill University, has conducted numerous studies on the effects of hormones on cognitive function, especially in older women. These and other studies have shown that estrogen replacement therapy reduces the incidence of Alzheimer's disease in older women.

Progesterone

Progesterone rebuilds bone, aids in the body's defense against cancer, decreases water retention to maintain proper weight, and promotes relaxation and better sleep.

Testosterone

Testosterone enhances endurance and coordination and produces a healthy libido, healthy hair, and a sense of security and safety, and supports drive, ambition, and focus. Testosterone is made in the testes of a man and the adrenals of a woman. Testosterone influences our ability to think in certain ways. Men and women who have better spatial memory have higher testosterone levels. Examples include an enhanced ability to handle tools or superior rhythm and dancing abilities. Testosterone fortifies the muscles, arteries, and nerves, including those in the brain.

Thierry Hertoghe, MD, a specialist in hormone balancing, explains that "when testosterone is low the arteries in the brain weaken, growing too soft in some places and increasing the risk of blood clots and stroke while growing too stiff in others and increasing the risk of high blood pressure and cerebral hemorrhage."[31]

Imbalance Challenges

Our sex hormones can become imbalanced for a number of reasons:

Chronic stress

Eating a diet high in sugar, refined carbs, and bad fats

Excessive alcohol consumption

Exposure to environmental toxins

Smoking

Symptoms of Sex Hormone Imbalance

The symptoms of sex hormone imbalance in women are these:

Estrogen deficiency reveals itself as hot flashes, trouble falling asleep, headaches and migraines, weight gain, warm rushes, vaginal dryness, mental fogginess, intestinal bloating, back and joint pain, temperature swings, racing mind at night, depression, and heart palpitations.

Progesterone deficiency reveals itself through difficulty sleeping, no period, frequent and heavy periods, cystic breasts, anxiety and nervousness, infrequent periods, spotting before periods, painful breasts, water retention, shorter cycle, premenstrual syndrome (PMS), endometriosis, and fibroids.

Testosterone deficiency reveals itself through diminished sex drive, diminished energy and stamina, diminished coordination and balance, flabbiness, diminished sense of security, indecisiveness, hair loss, and muscle weakness.

Pregnenolone

Pregnenolone has been referred to as the "memory hormone" because of its astounding ability to improve memory. Pregnenolone is the most abundant hormone in the brain and is concentrated about seventy-five times more in the brain than in the blood. Pregnenolone helps the short-term memory cells sprout in the part of the brain called the hippocampus. The hippocampus is the area deep inside your brain where your sense of "self" lives. I like to think of pregnenolone as the mother hormone, because it is the building block from which a number of other hormones are created, including estrogen, testosterone, progesterone, and DHEA.[32]

In fact, a study on those with a mental illness called *schizoaffective disorder* showed improvement in memory and attention after just eight weeks of taking 30 mg of pregnenolone a day.[33] Whenever you are self-dosing with hormones that do not need a medical prescription, such as DHEA and pregnenolone, you have to be careful of taking too much, as higher levels of these hormones in the blood can flood the receptor sites, which then downregulate, rendering the hormone no longer effective. It's a bit like overwatering a plant—you can damage a plant if you flood the root system and the excess water has nowhere to drain. If you are taking this hormone, I strongly recommend you work with your doctor or become one of my patients in order to have your blood levels monitored once every few months.

Thyroid Hormone

Thyroid hormone has significant effects upon thought processes and memory, in large part because it helps optimize blood flow. When thyroid hormone levels are low, people often complain of feeling cold, because their blood flow is reduced, their uptake of oxygen is diminished, and the number of connections between the brain cells is decreased. Just a small amount of improved physiological levels of thyroid hormone can help someone's mental focus tremendously, as well as assist with depression.

Your thyroid gland is located in your neck just above your larynx (voice box). It controls the rate at which almost all your biochemical reactions occur. If your thyroid function is slow and out of balance, every part of your body and brain will be slow and out of balance.

Thyroid hormone is also the single most important hormone that enables your body to efficiently use oxygen. Therefore, if your thyroid gland is not producing enough thyroid hormone, or if you are unable to convert inactive thyroid hormone into the active form, or if the receptor sites for thyroid hormone are blocked, then you can feel like you just don't have enough oxygen or life force.

Here are the most common symptoms of a low-functioning thyroid:

Constipation

Cracked and chipping fingernails

Depression

Dry skin and dry hair

Fatigue

Fluid retention

Hair loss

Insomnia

Low sex drive

Memory loss

Menstrual problems

Muscle aches and cramps

Premenstrual syndrome

Sluggishness

Trouble getting up in the morning

Weight gain

Many people today suffer from thyroid issues, but why is this? Using four iodine molecules from our diet, the thyroid gland produces the thyroid hormone thyroxine (T4). T4 is an inactive form of thyroid. This thyroid hormone, T4, is then converted into triiodothyronine (T3) by a certain enzyme that is on the kidney and liver. About a third of the T4 is converted into the active form, T3, another third is converted to an inactive form, rT3, and the latter third is broken down to be eliminated by the body. The central nervous system, pituitary, and brown fat tissue help maintain T3 as the active hormone. This is why, when a person suffers a brain injury, the damage can affect the circulation going to their pituitary gland and central nervous system, thereby producing less T3. The conversion of T4 to T3 requires the presence of several nutrients: selenium, vitamin A, vitamin D, and zinc. A key issue causing thyroid problems is deficiencies in these nutrients, as well as in iodine. You can refer back to chapter 3, "Nourishing Your Brain," to learn more about these nutrients.

Thyroid-Toxic Chemicals

A second major issue that can cause poor thyroid function is toxins. Toxins that can damage the thyroid are pathogens (such as infection by a virus or bacteria), heavy metals, food allergens, and environmental toxins, such as PCBs and industrial petrochemicals.

Bromide (which is found in bromated water or flour) blocks iodine uptake.

Chlorine blocks iodine uptake by the thyroid gland. When you take a shower or a bath, any chlorine in the water is absorbed through your skin.

Fluoride in your drinking water, shower, and bath blocks iodine uptake by the thyroid gland. I highly recommend you use a water filter for your shower or bath to take out both chlorine and fluoride. A good affordable brand is Rainshow'r.

To fully assess thyroid function, it's helpful to have a full panel of thyroid lab tests, including both inactive T4 and active T3 hormone, TSH, thyroid antibodies, nutrient levels, heavy metal levels, food allergies, and the presence of either viruses or pathogenic bacteria.

Stress Hormones

Our stress hormones are created by our two adrenal glands, which are small triangular organs that sit on top of the kidneys. These glands secrete adrenaline, which supports our ability to "get up and go." Each adrenal gland has an inner central area called the medulla and an outer cortex. The inner part makes pregnenolone and DHEA, which help with neuroplasticity, that is, the fluidity of the brain—its ability to adapt to change, increase its synaptic connections, and give us energy. The outer part of the adrenal gland makes cortisol, epinephrine, and norepinephrine, which enhance our energy in the same way caffeine does.

There are three major stages of stress that affect our stress hormone production:

Stage I is when the pituitary gland sends out large amounts of adrenocorticotropic hormone (ACTH), which stimulates the production of cortisol. Elevated cortisol inhibits serotonin, T3, and DHEA production; it also decreases insulin sensitivity, which leads to blood sugar issues.

Stage II occurs when a prolonged period of stress causes an even higher demand for cortisol. ACTH production remains high as the pituitary gland continues to signal the adrenals to stay "on." At this point, sex hormone imbalances also begin to take place.

Stage III, also known as adrenal fatigue, happens when there is very low cortisol, DHEA, epinephrine, and norepinephrine, and the person feels exhausted all the time. Even worse, since we need healthy levels of stress hormones to make melatonin (the hormone that helps you sleep), these people can't sleep even though they are exhausted.

Melatonin and Sleep

One out of every three Americans is sleep deprived.[34] You don't have to be one of them. Almost all of us need seven to eight hours of sleep a night. One of the first steps to take if you are experiencing poor memory is to **allow yourself to get eight hours of sleep a night for two weeks in a row**. Then see if your memory improves. Sleeping is the single most important thing you can do to achieve long-term mental and physical health. A lack of sleep can lead to depression, chronic pain, heart disease, obesity, and fatigue. During sleep, melatonin is produced by the pineal gland, provided that your bedroom is sufficiently dark. The melatonin also acts as a brain antioxidant.

While we are sleeping, our brain repairs itself. In fact, the brain actually shrinks 60 percent at night when we are sleeping. Just like the ocean, in which the tide recedes and then comes forward, the fluid around the brain recedes into the body during sleep. This "ebb" of fluid flushes out the harmful tau protein, amyloid plaques, and other toxins, which in turn helps lower the risk of dementia.

Here is a great Ted Talk on the importance of sleep.[35]

The Effect of Insulin on Your Body and Brain

In addition to the negative effects of imbalances in cortisol, adrenaline, and thyroid hormone, one of the most common and debilitating hormonal issues in our country is excessive insulin resulting from the consumption of too many simple sugars. Over 100 million Americans are diagnosed with a condition called *insulin resistance* as a result of their diet and lifestyle. Excessive insulin levels not only increase the chances of heart attack, kidney failure, and a decreased life span, they also increase our likelihood of getting dementia by crippling our blood circulation.

Insulin is the chemical that escorts sugar into our cells, where it is transformed into energy. Insulin resistance occurs especially when we eat too many simple sugars, when we don't exercise, when we experience too much stress, and when we don't get adequate sleep at night. Under these conditions your body will pump out more insulin than your cells require.

The summary below is according to a study in 2013 from the *Journal of Endocrinology of Metabolic Clinics of North America*:

> *Today's "around the clock" society, characterized by demands for high work performance, prolonged daily commutes, and less leisure activity, has significantly compromised sleep duration. Self-reported sleep times have decreased from over 8 hours in the 1960s to approximately 6.5 hours in 2012. Up to 30% of middle-aged Americans sleep less than six hours a night. Similar results were reported in other countries and were confirmed in population-based cohorts where sleep duration was objectively measured. Sleep duration is also compromised by sleep disorders such as insomnia and obstructive sleep apnea. Whether it is voluntarily or involuntarily compromised, sleep loss has significant health consequences. These consequences range from impaired cognitive function to increased all-cause morbidity and mortality. Derangements in sleep also affect glucose homeostasis and appetite control. Impaired sleep thus might contribute to the rising prevalence of type 2 diabetes (T2DM) and obesity in modern society.*[36]

Lack of sleep can lead to more insulin resistance, in which your cells develop a tolerance to insulin. The receptor sites for insulin in your cells become resistant to it. The insulin that is not accepted into the cell ends up floating around in your blood. Over time, a set of symptoms can occur, which often include these:

A fat belly

High blood pressure

High triglycerides

Inflammation in your blood

Low levels of high-density lipoproteins (HDL)

Slightly higher blood sugar levels

This complex list of health problems is known as *metabolic syndrome* and can lead to pre-dementia. At high levels, insulin acts as a major fat-storage hormone and creates mood and behavior disturbances; it also increases bad cholesterol (low-density lipoprotein, or LDL) while lowering good cholesterol (high-density lipoprotein, or HDL) and increasing appetite. Too much insulin can raise blood pressure and stimulate the growth of cancer cells. It can increase inflammation and oxidative stress, as well as age the brain and cause sex hormone problems.

Here are two supplements to manage elevated insulin:

Alpha lipoic acid (ALA), 600 mg taken three times a day can lower blood glucose levels by helping the liver manage insulin resistance. It acts similarly to the drug metformin. Scientific studies have also supported its use for diabetic neuropathy.

Chromium at levels of 1,000 mcg per day enhances the activity of insulin at the cellular level. At 200 mcg per day it also helps people with blood glucose swings and sugar and starch cravings. These recommended doses have been backed by double-blind controlled trials.

Basic Plan for Balancing Hormones

Let's begin with the nutritional steps I recommend for restoring your hormones to proper balance. Note that some of these recommendations overlap with my earlier general recommendations.

Cut Out All Simple Sugars from Your Diet

When attempting to cut out all simple sugars from your diet, it's useful to know why. For example, just one teaspoon of sugar (most soda drinks have five teaspoons) impairs the immune system's ability to fight infection for up to six hours. As we have noted, sugar is the number one contributing factor to insulin resistance, a symptom of metabolic syndrome. By *simple sugars*, I am referring to foods that contain cane sugar, honey, high-fructose corn syrup (in foods like ketchup, salad dressings, breakfast cereals, and sauces in restaurants), all other forms of fructose (found in most health-food bars and drinks), and syrups. Also, fruit juices should be avoided. Whole fruit is okay because the fiber in whole fruit helps the sugar get digested and absorbed by the intestinal system slowly. For a sugar substitute, green stevia is one alternative. Keeping your blood sugar even throughout the day helps the adrenal glands tremendously. Remember, you get the sugar you need from the breakdown of healthy carbohydrates such as whole fruits and vegetables.

Increase Your Fiber Intake to Twenty-Five Grams a Day

Fiber is essential for healthy gut bacteria, also known as our *microbiome*. In the last few years, we have witnessed an exciting influx of research on the gut microbiome and its multitude of effects on mood, weight, the bowels, and much more. Believe it or not, in our body we have ten times more DNA that comes from bacteria than from human cells! Among many other things, these gut bacteria are *neurotrophic*; that is,

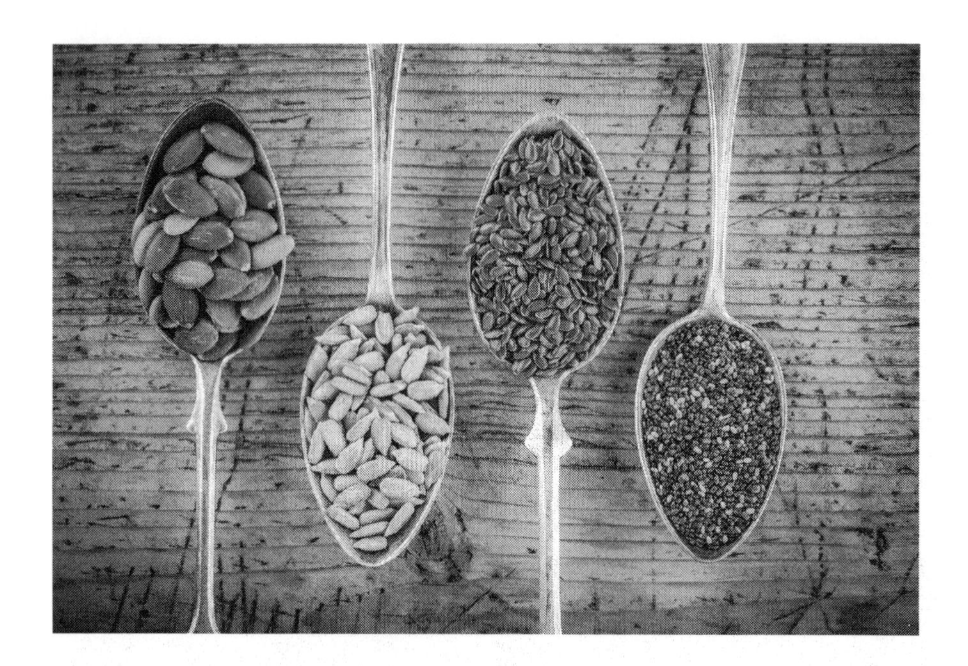

they grow nerves. They stimulate BDNF, as we discussed previously, as well as many related factors in the neurological system that can help with focus, attention, and memory.

It's actually quite challenging to get 25 g of fiber (my daily recommendation) from food alone, so you may need to supplement with chia seeds or freshly ground flaxseed. Fiber not only feeds our microbiome, it also slows down our digestion, thereby balancing our blood sugar. That's why fruit is best eaten with its skin and pulp, rather than taken as juice.

Ingest Other Hormone-Friendly Nutrients

Here is a list of other hormone-friendly nutrients:

Dandelion greens are rich in vitamin A.

Fish has omega-3 fats and vitamin D, as well as iodine.

Seaweed, dulse flakes, and kelp powder or tincture have iodine for your thyroid.

Smelt, herring, scallops, and Brazil nuts have selenium.

Avoid Toxic Foods and Substances

Certain foods must be avoided because they can cause an immune reaction, which creates antibodies that attack the thyroid. Some people have what's called gluten sensitivity. When a person eats foods that contain gluten, they can get inflammation in their gut lining, giving them gas, bloating, nausea, and difficulty digesting. Many people believe that because they have gas, bloating, and difficulty with their bowel movements, they have celiac disease; however, this is not always the case.

A recently published study in the journal *Digestion* (June 11, 2015) found that 86 percent of individuals who believed they were gluten sensitive could tolerate gluten.[37] Individuals with celiac disease, a hereditary autoimmune condition that affects about three million Americans, or roughly 1 percent of the population, must avoid gluten. If you have celiac disease, which is diagnosed either by a biopsy of the small intestine, performed by a gastroenterologist, or by a blood test, then even a small amount of gluten, say the size of a crouton, can cause inflammation of the gut lining for up to three months! For people who have gluten sensitivity or celiac disease, foods to avoid are bread and flour products, wheat, barley, rye, oats, spelt, and processed soy.

If you don't know if you have gluten sensitivity or celiac disease, you can cut out those foods for at least two weeks in a row and see if you feel different. If you are truly sensitive, usually you have a lot more mental clarity, feel like you have more energy, and may lose weight when you cut those foods out. If you do feel a big difference, it's a good idea to get tested by your doctor for celiac disease.

Balance Hormonal Health with Botanicals

Mother Nature has provided us with an armamentarium of plant medicine that can help us. Unlike pharmaceuticals, in which one drug has a very specific function based on a particular biochemical reaction, plant medicine (also referred to as herbs) helps modulate several functions in the body. In fact, most pharmaceuticals actually come from studying plants and extracting their medicinal components. Out of 118 drugs, 74 percent **come from plants**, 18 percent from fungi, 5 percent from bacteria, and 3 percent from vertebrate species such as snakes or frogs.[38]

Adaptogenic herbs in particular increase our resilience to high demands on our physical energy and mental rigor. They support our learning, mental sharpness, and acuity. I cannot cover the full scope of plant medicine in this book; however, I can share with you four key herbal botanicals for the brain: St. John's wort, ginkgo, rhodiola, and bacopa.

St. John's wort

When I first realized that I had many of the symptoms of ADD from my bicycle accident at age fourteen, I read a book called *Healing ADD: The Breakthrough Program That Allows You to See and Heal the 6 Types of ADD* (2002) by Daniel G. Amen, MD, a psychiatrist. That revolutionized my thinking around how a physically traumatic blow to the brain can cause damage to my ability to focus and feel calm. His book led me to taking St. John's wort, and to be honest, after three days of taking it, I felt as though my racing mind had slowed down tenfold. I wondered how just taking a couple of capsules of this herb a day could have such a powerful effect on my ability to stay focused and to feel less sad. My mood lifted almost miraculously. That's because St. John's wort (*Hypericum perforatum*) acts as a mild antidepressant.

St John's wort is a botanical plant that has antibacterial, antiviral, anticancer, antioxidant, neuroprotective, and anti-inflammatory properties. The active constituents of St. John's wort, hyperforin and adhyperforin, inhibit the reuptake, as well as modulate the effects, of serotonin, dopamine, and norepinephrine. In most studies of individuals with depression or anxiety, St. John's wort at 300 mg three times a day performed just as well as the SSRI or standard antidepressant medications, except without the side effects.[39]

Rhodiola

Rhodiola (*Rhodiola rosea*) is a wonderful plant that thrives in cold regions and high altitudes and is notorious for its ability to increase resistance to physical, chemical, and biological stressors. In vitro and animal studies have shown the constituents rhodioloside, salidroside, and tyrosol regulate the activity of serotonin, dopamine, and norepinephrine, as well as inhibit monoamine oxidase A (MAO-A).

Ginkgo biloba

The popular herbal plant for memory *Ginkgo biloba* is featured in the cover image of my book. Ginkgo comes from one of the oldest species of trees in the world. This tree is called the maidenhair tree and can grow more than 130 feet tall and live for over 1,000 years. Some trees in China are said to be over 2,500 years old. In fact, this tree is considered to be a living fossil, meaning that it continues to survive even after major extinction events. Research studies have shown that it improves memory, thinking, and the ability to perform everyday tasks, and that an extract of ginkgo (called EGb 761) was clinically effective in treating Alzheimer's. There are high levels of flavonoids, terpenoids, and antioxidants in ginkgo that promote blood circulation in the brain and protect other parts of the brain from neuronal damage.[40]

Bacopa

The herb *Bacopa monnieri* is considered a nootropic, which means that it boosts cognitive function in the short term while supporting long-term brain health. Bacopa has been used for centuries in the ancient Indian healing branch of Ayurveda. Bacopa outperformed ginseng and a standard medication called Provigil used to create alertness in people who have a sleeping disorder. It also helped the most with verbal word recall. The benefits of bacopa can be attributed to a group of triterpenoid saponins called *bacosides*. Bacopa provides several key support pathways for the brain: neuroprotection, communication between brain cells, neuromodulation and adaptation to stress, reducing beta-amyloid accumulation, and enhancing blood flow. The bacosides in bacopa have been shown in rodent studies to bolster important antioxidants in the brain: catalase, superoxide dismutase, and glutathione. Bacopa increases the branching of neurons into more pathways for memory and cognitive clarity in the brain. They create more synapses for dendrites. Bacopa also raises acetylcholine levels in the brain, which in turn helps with memory and concentration. It does this by inhibiting the function of acetylcholinesterase, an enzyme that normally breaks down acetylcholine. Last but not least, bacopa helps improve circulation in the brain through vasodilation of the blood vessels by increasing nitric oxide, a substance that helps with opening up the flow of blood (the same way Viagra works for erectile dysfunction).

There are some impressive research studies on bacopa:

- A group of adults took either *Bacopa monnieri* or a placebo for at least twelve weeks. Those who took bacopa experienced a consistently reduced reaction time and speed compared with those who didn't.[41]
- A second study showed that within hours of taking the herb, multitasking performance was improved and anxiety was reduced during cognitively demanding tasks.[42]

When taking bacopa, look for a source that is 55% bacosides by weight. You can take 300 mg once a day with food. Store it in a cool, dark place.

Ashwagandha

Ashwagandha (*Withania somnifera*) has long been used in the traditional Ayurvedic system of medicine to enhance memory and improve cognition. In a study on fifty adults, improvement in executive function, sustained attention, and information-processing speed occurred after only eight weeks of taking ashwagandha.[43]

With all botanical medicines, you need to be aware that they may interfere with the processes of other pharmaceuticals you are on and that you must stop taking them one week prior to surgery. The quality of herbal medicine varies greatly, and you want to use only the brands that your doctor recommends. I personally rely on an herbal company that has to follow *United States Pharmacopeia* pharmaceutical standards and whose laboratory I have visited in order to witness their quality-control standards.

Bioidentical Hormone Replacement

As I have noted, hormones interact directly with the brain and affect mood and cognition. Occasionally getting hormone therapy from your doctor can be both lifesaving and "brain-saving." Most of my patients feel like a new person within three days of hormone therapy. One patient, a therapist who was writing a book on emotional health, told me "I had no idea one could feel this good. This is the best I've felt in thirty years!"

Bioidentical hormone replacement therapy (BHRT), also known as *bioidentical hormone therapy* or *natural hormone therapy*, is the use of hormones that are identical on a molecular level to endogenous hormones (produced by the human body). BHRT is not the same as taking Premarin or Prempro, which have synthetic hormones from the urine of a pregnant horse. Synthetic hormones have received a reputation for increasing the chances of heart attack, stroke, pulmonary embolism, and breast cancer, and the medical field was encouraged to stop prescribing hormones for women past menopause. BHRT can be derived from plants instead of from the urine of a pregnant horse; thus, it is more bioidentical at a molecular level.

Why consider taking bioidentical hormones over the regular Premarin or Prempro? The Women's Health Initiative (WHI) was undertaken over a 14-year time span, from 1991 to 2005, on 16,000 women aged 50 to 79. The results were published in *The Journal of the American Medical Association* and a follow-up was carried out later, for a total of 18 years. This study summarized comprehensively over 117 different publications and a wealth of WHI data on overall health risks and benefits of hormone therapy for postmenopausal women. Because it showed a 20 to 30 percent relative risk increase in breast cancer occurring with estrogen and progesterone therapy, physicians dramatically pulled back on prescribing hormones. There was more to the story. When the study is viewed in more detail, it shows that there was a 20 percent decrease in breast cancer with estrogen therapy alone. It actually was the synthetic progesterone used in the study that increased the cancer risk.

Uzzi Reiss, MD, OB/GYN, in his book *Natural Hormone Balance*, says

> *A qualitative review of 90% of the world literature from 1975–2000 to assess whether recent epidemiological evidence supports an association between the use of estrogen replacement therapy or hormone replacement therapy and breast cancer was performed. The tabulated results of 50 epidemiological and 6 meta-analysis studies concluded the following:*
>
> *Estrogen users are less likely to die from breast cancer than non-users.*
>
> *Cancers associated with hormone use are often less aggressive, less metastatic, so hormones may modulate the tumor in some way.*

Hormones that are bioidentical can be ingested in the form of oral capsules, cheek lozenges, drops, creams, vaginal suppositories, or injectable testosterone for men. Taking such substances requires a prescription, so they require a visit to a physician's office, as well as monitoring the levels on an annual or semiannual basis. The women I place on bioidentical hormones are almost always extremely grateful for the inherent difference in how they feel while on them.

Lab Work

These are the laboratory tests I recommend to check for a healthy balance in your hormone levels.

For Insulin Balance, Inflammation, and Healthy Fat Levels

A two-hour glucose tolerance test measuring insulin and glucose may be needed to determine your insulin balance. Additional lab tests to check for blood glucose, inflammation, and cholesterol levels are these:

HbA1C to measure the amount of glucose in your system for the past three months

Fasting cholesterol profile

C-RP to check for inflammation in the body

Liver function tests such as GGT, AST, and ALT to assess for fatty liver

Thyroid Balance

To determine a person's thyroid balance, most doctors only order the test for thyroid stimulating hormone (TSH). This is inadequate, because sometimes the TSH level can be normal while the thyroid hormones are not. I have seen this often in my clinical practice. A healthy pituitary responds by producing TSH when blood thyroid levels are low. If the pituitary is unhealthy, however, it can respond suboptimally and give a TSH level that looks normal but actually would be high if the pituitary were healthier. A history of brain injury can create a suboptimal pituitary function for years to come.

What you really need to see are the results of these tests:

Anti-thyroglobulin antibodies

Free T3

Free T4

Reverse T3

Thyroid peroxidase (TPO)

TSH

Testing Your Sex Hormones

These tests can be done by sampling blood, saliva, or urine:

DHEA-S

Free testosterone

Pregnenolone

Progesterone

Sex hormone binding globulin (SHBG)

Total estrogens (can be broken down into free estradiol, estrone, and estriol).

5 | HEALING LEAKY GUT AND LEAKY BRAIN

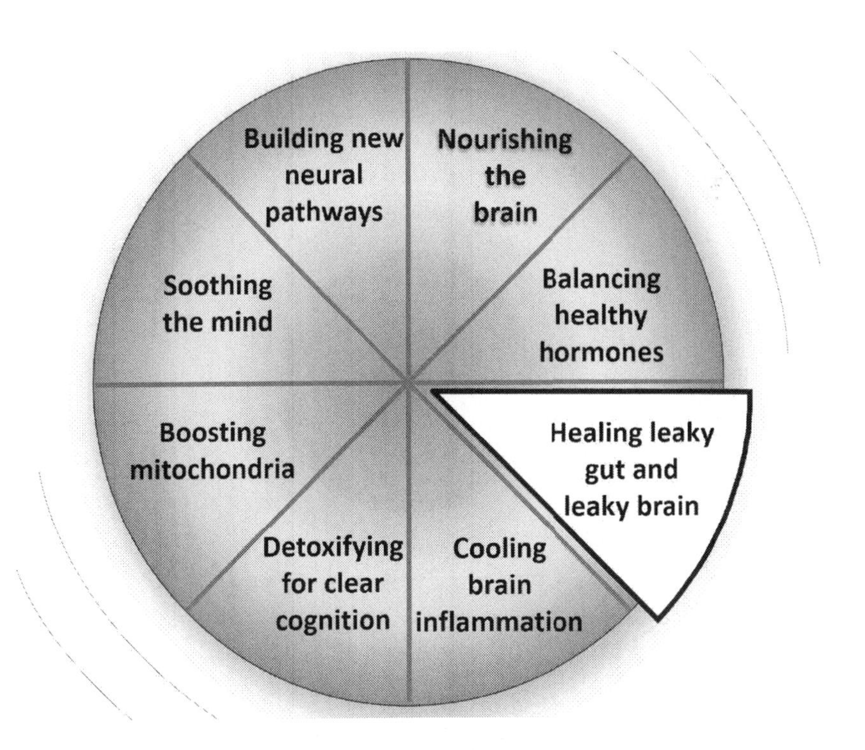

What do the brain and the gut have in common? The answer is the structure of the blood-brain barrier (BBB) and the gut lining. Often ignored because of their seemingly unimpressive anatomy, these two are highly crucial to our health. The BBB is a highly selective semipermeable border that separates the circulating blood from the brain and extracellular fluid in the central nervous system (CNS). The BBB may become leaky in select neurological diseases. Our intestines have a similarly important lining that acts as a sieve. This is from an article published in the US National Library of Medicine, National Institutes of Health:

> *The intestinal epithelium is a single-cell layer that constitutes the largest and most important barrier against the external environment. It acts as a selectively permeable barrier permitting the absorption of nutrients, electrolytes and water, while maintaining an effective defense against intraluminal toxins, antigens and enteric flora.*[44]

Leaky gut leads to leaky brain. The gut leaks inflammatory products that then enter the defenseless brain through the weakened BBB and begin to activate the brain's immune system. The cells that make up this immune system are called *microglia*, because they are much smaller than the neural cells known as *glia*. Microglia form a glue around our neural cells. They are tiny cells with arms that stick out into the extracellular matrix (the tissue outside the cells), monitoring it for toxins or danger. Originally, they were derived from the bone marrow before arriving and staying in the brain, so their embryological origin is different from that of the brain and spinal cord. When healthy, microglia destroy plaque and remove dead cells. However, they can convert to inflammatory products and puff up to become larger cells, causing collateral damage and injury when they are exposed to insult, such as brain trauma. To fix the leaky brain, you must first fix the leaky gut. To understand more about the microglia and how inflammation in the brain can be a switch that turns on and stays on, watch this five-minute video on Khan Academy entitled *Microglia.*[45]

What we eat has a powerful physiological effect on our brain, which is understandable when you appreciate the nature of this lining in the intestines and in the brain. Many of my patients notice a significant improvement in their mental clarity when they change their diet. By eating in a way that keeps inflammation low in the gut, they are actually lowering inflammation in the brain. The tissue proteins making up the BBB are similar to the tissue proteins of the intestinal barrier. There are connections between the intestinal cells called *tight junctions*. They are tight for a reason: they keep the bigger food molecules out and let the smaller, fully digested molecules in. Picture a sieve with small holes. When we continue to eat inflammatory foods, these junctions enlarge. Another way to think of it is that the sieve holes get bigger. This is where the term "leaky gut" comes from. These larger food molecules that come through the widened junctions can become antigenic substances in your bloodstream. They are seen as foreign, and they ramp up the immune system reaction. The result is a delayed hypersensitivity food reaction, which can result in brain fog; lethargy; rash; swelling; skin changes like rough, dry skin patches, psoriasis, and eczema; or dark circles under the eyes.

If you suffer from either leaky gut or leaky brain, you need to repair both at the same time. Since the immune system does not establish tolerance to brain antigens, when there is a breakdown of the BBB, destruction of neurological tissues occurs quickly. Breakdown in the BBB is thought to play a role in multiple disorders, including Alzheimer's, Parkinson's, traumatic brain injury, multiple sclerosis, AIDS dementia, amyotrophic lateral sclerosis, and epilepsy.

A study published in the *Lancet* found subjects with inflammatory bowel disease developed white-matter lesion in the brain, as identified by magnetic resonance imaging (MRI), with almost the same frequency as patients with multiple sclerosis (a disease of brain myelin destruction). In fact, 42 percent of patients with Crohn's disease and 46 percent of patients with ulcerative colitis have white matter lesions in their brains.[46] Another shocking statistic that supports the link between the inflammation in the gut and in the brain is that 50 to 90 percent of those with irritable bowel syndrome also had panic disorder, post-traumatic stress disorder, generalized anxiety, and depression.

Causes of Leaky Gut

Many of us have heard of the negative effects of gluten, which comes from flour or wheat. Gluten from wheat can create opioid-like proteins that cause brain fog. Continued consumption of reactive foods such as gluten have the potential to create continual inflammation of your small intestine. Gluten isn't the only thing that can cause leaky gut. The following is a list of other causes:

Diet: alcohol, gluten, casein, processed foods with food coloring or preservatives, excess sugar, food allergies

Medications: corticosteroids, antibiotics, antacids, xenobiotics

Infections: *Helicobacter pylori* (*H. pylori*), bacterial overgrowth, yeast overgrowth, intestinal virus, parasitic infection

Hormonal: decreased levels of thyroid hormone, testosterone, estrogen, or progesterone

Stress: increased cortisol

Neurologic: brain trauma, stroke, neurodegeneration

Metabolic: glycosylated end products, intestinal inflammation, autoimmune conditions

Glyphosate: a pesticide used in agriculture, which can be in our drinking water and food

Just by reading this, you may already have a sense of what physical health issues you have that are affecting your brain, from diet, hormones, stress, brain trauma, and now possibly leaky gut.

Herbicide: Glyphosate Is Also Known as Roundup

One issue that is insidious and yet ubiquitous is that of glyphosate from genetically modified organisms (GMO). I'd like to take a moment here to go into glyphosate a little more.

"Although there are many toxins that impair mitochondrial function, one of the most prevalent is glyphosate (used in Roundup). Roundup suppresses mitochondrial complexes II and III, which are a crucial part of the electron transport chain function. The Environmental Working Group has found the degradation product of glyphosate in 75 percent of air and rain samples near the Mississippi Delta farmlands in 2007."[47] This cellular energy, ATP, is responsible for physical and mental energy.

Roundup, or glyphosate, is one of the most toxic herbicides or insecticides tested. Exposure to glyphosate has been linked to autism, Alzheimer's, anxiety, cancer, depression, fatigue, gluten sensitivity, inflammation, and Parkinson's. The effects of glyphosate on the body have been ignored by the medical profession. Fortunately, one individual, Jeffrey Smith, an American activist, best-selling author, and movie director, began studying the effects of glyphosate at great depth before anyone else, scouring years of data. Jeffrey Smith is the founding director of the Institute of Responsible Technology and has been educating the world for the past twenty-two years on GMOs, Roundup, and their perilous health effects, lecturing in forty-five different countries, writing books, and being interviewed in movies. Watch the movies *OMG-GMO: Is This the End of Real Food* and *Secret Ingredients* to fully comprehend the extent of this issue.

Beginning in the 1990s, the genetic modification of organisms is a process in which a gene from a virus or bacteria is forced into the gene of another species. The FDA reviewed GMOs in the 1990s and said there needed to be further studies on possible toxicity due to new allergens forming in Monsanto's genetically modified food. For example, genetically modified corn produces cadaverine and putrescine, the chemicals that make a cadaver stink, and genetically modified soy is seven times more allergenic than regular soy. The person in charge of policy at the FDA, however, became the vice president of Monsanto while still working for the FDA, and the scrutiny on GMOs was lifted. The list of genetically modified foods currently consists of soy, corn, cotton, cottonseed oil, canola, zucchini, apples, potatoes, sugar beets, alfalfa (hay), papaya from China or Hawaii, and salmon.

GMOs are also in the animals that we feed with those foods, such as corn-fed beef. Interestingly, both animals and humans have the same diseases, which are rising with the use of GMOs. Animals that ate genetically modified feed were found to have early death, precancerous cells, multiple tumors, small brains, and shrunken livers and testicles.

Jeffrey Smith compiled data to look at the diseases associated with GMOs, and they are these:

Digestive problems 85%
Fatigue 60%
Overweight or obesity 54%
Brain fog 51%
Mood issues such as anxiety and depression 51%
Food allergies 50%
Poor memory and concentration 48%
Joint pain 47%
Seasonal allergies 46%
Gluten sensitivities 42%
Insomnia 33%
Skin conditions other than eczema 30%
Hormonal problems 30%
Musculoskeletal pain 25%
Autoimmune disease 21%
Eczema 21%
Cardiovascular problems 20%
High blood pressure 19%
Asthma 14%
Menstrual problems 13%

Diabetes 10%
Mental disorders other than depression and anxiety 7.9%
Underweight 6.5%
Cancer 4.8%
Kidney disease 4.5%
Infertility 3.8%
Autism spectrum 2%
Alzheimer's 2%
Parkinson's disease 1%

Studies by the American Academy of Environmental Medicine show that these diseases also appear in animals, and that animals get better when they are taken off genetically modified foods, just as humans do.

In order to understand the physiological effects of genetically modified food, we have to also learn about Roundup. Roundup is an herbicide that is put on genetically modified crops to kill weeds. Genetically modified crops are "Roundup ready," meaning that they are immune to Roundup. Roundup is also known as glyphosate, and it was used initially to clean boilers by stripping away the mineral buildup in pipes. Roundup is sprayed on genetically modified crops heavily three to five days prior to harvest. Glyphosate is a mitochondrial toxin—it disrupts key physiological mechanisms.

Yet another physiological process that GMOs block, which can cause mood issues and ADHD, is the shikimate pathway in plants. What this means is that the genetically modified plants we eat can't create the essential amino acids we need to help our mood. Glyphosate works by inhibiting the synthesis of tryptophan, phenylalanine, and tyrosine in plants. Interestingly, humans need these three amino acids to make our appropriate happy or peaceful brain chemistry. When food sources have scarce amounts of these amino acids due to glyphosate use, humans are at risk of deficiency too.

Glyphosate breaks down the BBB, leading to a leaky gut/brain axis, because it decreases the number of good bacteria in the gut, such as *Bifidobacteria* and *Lactobacilli.* Glyphosate allows for the overgrowth of harmful bacteria such as *Campylobacter* and *Clostridium difficile.*

An article titled "Roundup Linked to Global Boom in Celiac Disease and Gluten Intolerance" stated,

> *Celiac disease, gluten intolerance and irritable bowel syndrome are on the rise worldwide, and that rise has taken place in parallel with the increased use of glyphosate (Roundup) herbicide, shows a new US peer-reviewed paper from Dr. Anthony Samsel and Dr. Stephanie Seneff. The review has been published in the* Journal of Interdisciplinary Toxicology.[48]

It's interesting that as the rates of GMOs and Roundup use have gone up in our food supply, we find two terrible conditions in our pediatric population: cancer and autism. Cancer is the number one killer in kids today, and the autism rate that was 1 out of 10,000 in the 80s is now up to 1 out of 27.

Glyphosate is a probable carcinogen in humans, and possible cancers linked to glyphosate exposure include non-Hodgkin's lymphoma, renal tubule carcinoma, pancreatic islet cell adenoma, and skin tumors. Studies have also indicated that glyphosate disrupts the microbiome in the intestine, causing a decrease in the ratio of beneficial to harmful bacteria. Renal tubular nephropathy has reached epidemic proportions among young male farm workers in El Salvador, Nicaragua, Costa Rica, India, and Sri Lanka. Researchers propose that glyphosate forms stable chelates with a variety of toxic metals and some can be absorbed through the skin.[49]

Wouldn't you want to know if you had this horrible stuff in your system? This is tricky because glyphosate gets stored in our bones, our kidneys, intestine, and spleen. The Great Plains Lab is the only lab certified under the Clinical Laboratory Improvement Amendments of 1988 (CLIA) currently performing a test for glyphosate in the urine. In fact, I just saw a patient last week who has had gas, bloating, and diarrhea every time he eats wheat, as well as profuse allergies now for a couple years, and as a young father, he wanted to be checked out for wheat allergies so that he can remain healthy for his daughter. We were shocked to see that his blood test showed no allergens to wheat, but his glyphosate test was positive. Aside from giving him the non-GMO shopping guide, I am trying a new product shown to remove glyphosate from the intestines.

The good news is you can avoid GMOs, and people do get better when they stop eating genetically modified foods. The two best ways to avoid GMOs is to drink reverse osmosis water and to eat organic, non-GMO foods. People eating organic food have considerably lower concentrations of glyphosate in their urine. In Jeffrey Smith's travels, he found that when people were placed on a non-GMO diet they got better, as did animals. Fortunately, there is a health product on the market that has been scientifically shown in a research study to lower inflammation linked with glyphosate in the gut by up to 75 percent in just six weeks. The name of this supplement is Biome Medic, which you can get access to by using a link that comes with a discount code in the resources section at the end of this book. Biome Medic is specifically formulated to heal the gut microbiome from the effects of glyphosate. It both chelates and expels toxins while simultaneously feeding the gut with vital minerals and prebiotics to support the regeneration of the microvilli and aerobic bacteria colonies.

The Power of Your Intestinal Microbiome

We are all familiar with the expression "follow your gut." The gut has its very own neurotransmitters. In fact, every class of neurotransmitter found in your brain is also found in your gut, including serotonin,

95 percent of which resides in your gut. The intestinal microbiome is closely involved in the enteric nervous system, with bidirectional communication through the vagus nerve. This is why the cliché "follow your gut" has some validity, because our gut's nervous system is actually linked to our brain. The chemicals produced in the gut modulate the activity of the vagus nerve, which sends signals back up to the brain. The brain interprets the signal from the vagus nerve and in turn directs us toward relaxation and digestion or shuts down digestion and amps up the energy for alarm, fight, or flee. Likewise, if you feel alarmed, the vagus nerve then communicates alarm to the gut lining, and that changes the chemicals that are produced in the gut to ones that create more stress.

Together, your intestinal bacteria are called your microbiome. In fact, the bacteria in your intestine produce not just serotonin (which I discussed in chapter 4, "Balancing Healthy Hormones") but also other neurotransmitters that help with mental focus and concentration, such as acetylcholine and dopamine, and some of the stress neurotransmitters, such as norepinephrine.

Given the intimate connection described above, it is not surprising that our gut can cause problems in our brain and our brain can cause problems in our gut.

Functions of a Healthy Microbiome

There are more than five hundred species of microbes in our intestinal tract, referred to collectively as the microbiome. The microbiome populates the surface of our gut, which has a surface area of approximately a hundred square meters but is only one cell layer thick. There are approximately four pounds of these bacteria in the average adult human, and they constitute ten times as much of our DNA as our own DNA do. In a strange way, we are more bacteria than we are human! This microbiome lives in symbiosis with us. When we give the microbiome a nice place to live in our gut lining, it returns the favor by helping our cells—including our brain cells—to function optimally.

Our microbiome does the following:

Communicates bidirectionally with our brain

Detoxifies poisons

Digests food

Keeps our pH balance normal

Makes vitamins

Produces energy for our intestinal cells

Produces neurotransmitters

Regulates cholesterol metabolism

Good bacteria in our microbiome have to compete for space with bad microbes, just as your lawn may have weeds such as dandelion competing with grass for the same turf; hence the term *turf wars*. As part of the Regenerate Your Brain Program, you may be encouraged to take a probiotic containing good microbes. Probiotics occur naturally in fermented foods such as sauerkraut, kimchi (also known as kim chee), kombucha, and yogurt.

Butyrate: Fertilizer for Both the Brain and Gut

One of the essential activities of bacteria is fermentation, which happens in our intestines. When we have a diet filled with good fiber from our fruits and vegetables, rice bran, chia, nuts, and ground flaxseed, these fibers provide food for our gut microbiome, and they produce short chain fatty acids in their fermentation process. The most famous of the short chain fatty acids is butyrate, which has been discovered to not only nourish our intestine wall cells and help digestive motility but also to enter our bloodstream and cross the BBB, where it can actually facilitate the production of brain derived neurotrophic factor. Our gut bacteria and how well they ferment thus have a direct effect on our ability to learn and form new memories. What if I told you that some of our gut bacteria have been found to actually raise our consciousness and that some do the opposite and increase the risk of schizophrenia or bipolar illness!

In fact, research shows the following:

- High levels of *Lachnospiraceae* and other butyrate producing bacteria were found in people with high conscientiousness.[50]
- Elevated levels of *Saccharomyces cerevisiae*, *Candida*, and/or *Toxoplasma gondii* are associated with neuropsychiatric conditions such as schizophrenia and bipolar disease.[51]
- A study was carried out on 55 human volunteers aged between 30 and 60 with mild depression and anxiety. After being placed on 3 billion colony-forming units (CFUs) of bacteria, they showed a 50% improvement in depression scoring, 36% improvement in anxiety, 49% improvement in global severity index, and 60% improvement in anger-hostility scores. They also showed a 13% decrease in urinary free cortisol, a hormonal measure of chronic stress. The probiotic group displayed reductions in self-blame and improvements in chronic stress.[52]

Undigested Gluteomorphins and Your Brain

Another threat to optimal brain performance may arise from inadequate digestion of gluten or casein, resulting in gluteomorphins. Gluteomorphins (a.k.a. gliadorphins) are unusual peptides that affect the same receptors on your cells that opium and morphine do. These peptides set off a reaction in your immune system that inhibits proper brain function.

Ocean Robbins, CEO of Food Revolution Network, wrote in an article published on October 4, 2019,[53]

> Gluten *is an umbrella name for proteins called prolamins (primarily glutenin and gliadin) found in wheat, rye, barley, and the lesser-known triticale). Wheat grains include wheat berries, durum, emmer, semolina, spelt, farina, farro, graham, KAMUT Khorasan wheat, and einkorn....*
>
> *Wheat, rye, barley, and triticale are in in many of the following products.*
>
> **Wheat**: *bread, pasta, baked goods, sauces, cereals, soups, roux (a mixture of flour with a fat-like oil or butter, used as a thickening agent for soups and sauces), salad dressings, soy sauces*
>
> **Rye**: *cereals, rye beer, rye bread (e.g., pumpernickel)*
>
> **Barley**: *malt, malt extracts, malt vinegar, beer, soups, food coloring, Brewer's yeast*
>
> **Triticale**: *cereals, pasta, breads*

One out of every five Americans and Europeans are now gluten free. However, being gluten free isn't for everyone, as wheat has some nutritional benefits that are good for you if your immune system is not affected by eating wheat.

Whole Wheat Provides a Number of Important Nutrients

Many gluten-containing whole grains, including wheat, have a lot of fiber. Researchers have found that the bran in whole wheat, in particular, contains a critical prebiotic fiber that boosts *Bifidobacteria* content within the gut, helping to relieve many gastrointestinal issues.

And there are other valuable nutrients in wheat, too. Even whole-wheat spaghetti, which is not exactly at the pinnacle of healthy eating, is a rich source of B vitamins, magnesium, phosphorus, zinc, copper, manganese, and selenium, as well as unsaturated fatty acids.

If you're going to eat flour products and you value your health, then it's wise to make sure they're 100 percent whole grain. To determine this, read legally mandated ingredient lists, not just front-of-package claims, as these aren't always substantiated. Some bread is touted as being "multi-grain," which just means it contains more than one type of grain. It doesn't mean that any of those grains are whole grains.

If you see any reference to wheat flour and you don't see "whole grain" or "whole wheat" on the actual ingredient list, then you can assume the product contains white (refined) flour, which is far less beneficial.

Sprouted grains—products made using grains that have just begun to sprout or germinate—are another 100 percent whole grain option. Sprouted grains are digested more slowly in your body and are, therefore, easier on your blood sugar levels and less likely to trigger food cravings. What's more, the process of sprouting grains increases the bioavailability of nutrients such as zinc, iron, folate, magnesium, vitamin C, and protein.

Lastly, if you need to go gluten free, you are probably substituting wheat flour with rice flour. Rice, unfortunately, can have a lot of arsenic in it. In a 2018 study in 11,353 people (55 of whom had been diagnosed with celiac disease), researchers found that the blood levels of those on a gluten-free diet (whether they had celiac or not) had more mercury, lead, and cadmium in their blood than people who did not avoid gluten.[54]

Basic Plan to Fix Your Gut

A gut-healing diet such as the one offered in this program combines dietary recommendations with supplements to assist in gut healing. Often a probiotic is helpful, but there are a few other supplements that can help heal the gut lining and ease digestion. A good starting place is to take a digestive enzyme with each meal for six months; it will have the specific enzymes (proteases, lipases, and amylases) that break down animal proteins, vegetable fibers, and fats.

Hydrochloric Acid Support

Many people think that the problem is having too much hydrochloric acid (HCL, also known as *stomach acid*), which may be true for some. Often, however, digestive problems occur because the stomach is not producing enough stomach acid, which can cause reflux and heartburn. With age, the stomach naturally produces less acid. In this case, acid-blocking medications compound the problem. Adequate stomach acid is needed to break down food and activate digestive enzymes. When taking HCL supplements, please be supervised by your doctor. Start with one capsule or tablet at the beginning of each meal. Increase the dose by one capsule per meal until you have a warm feeling in your stomach, then drop back down to the dose just before the warm feeling occurred.

A Special Probiotic

A basic probiotic supplement is necessary for this program to work. The healthy bacteria in the gut not only reduce inflammation in the gut lining, help with gut immunity, improve digestive function, and lower the uptake into the gut lining of toxins such as heavy metals, but also help produce BDNF, which helps the brain with focus and memory. A healthy gut supports a healthy mind.

Scientists at Pacific Northwest National Laboratory have demonstrated that boosted levels of *Lactobacillus* are directly linked to enhanced memory. Higher levels of GABA, which of course is produced by some species of gut bacteria, are also associated with better memory.[55]

One of the mainstays of the gut repair program is supplementing once or twice a day on an empty stomach with these microorganisms:

- *Saccharomyces boulardii*, 150–200 mg (3–5 billion)
- *Lactobacillus*, 25 billion

Regenerating Gut Diet Plan to Heal the Leaky Gut

To avoid the stress on your body of having low blood sugar—a primary aim of the Regenerate Your Brain Program—eat regularly, stabilize your blood sugar, and do not allow yourself to become overly hungry. If you have a healthy gut lining then you can continue to focus on a broad array of grains, vegetables, legumes, and fruits. However, if your lab tests reveal that you have a leaky gut, then you may need to go on a much more restricted diet. I refer my patients with a severe case of leaky gut to the "gut and psychology syndrome," or GAPS, diet, as originated by neurologist and physician Natasha Campbell-McBride, MD. This diet is much more extensive than what I have outlined below. The one below is a good place to start, without the immediate guidance of a health care professional trained in nutrition.

Foods to Avoid

The following foods have the potential to aggravate the gut and cause both inflammation and allergies. You don't have to be off these permanently, but only partially for anywhere from two weeks to six months, depending on your symptoms and the results of your lab work.

Alcohol

All sugars and sweeteners, even honey and agave

Canned foods

Dairy: milk, cream, cheese, butter, whey, and so on

Eggs and all foods that contain eggs, such as mayonnaise

Grains: barley, buckwheat, corn, oats, quinoa, rice, wheat

High-glycemic fruits: canned fruits, dried fruits, grapes, mango, pineapple, raisins, watermelon

Instant coffee, because many brands of instant coffee are contaminated with gluten

Lectins, found in nuts, beans, potatoes, tomatoes, eggplant, peppers, peanut oil, and peanut butter

Mushrooms

Processed foods

Soy products, including soy milk, soy protein, soy sauce, soy oil, tempeh, tofu, and so on

Foods to Eat

The "foods to avoid" list can look daunting, but there are many foods you can eat. You will begin to feel so good after a while that you will enjoy eating this way. Once the gut lining is healed, you can slowly reintroduce the foods from the foods-to-avoid list.

Here is a list of foods that you can eat:

Coconut: coconut oil, coconut butter, coconut milk, coconut cream, coconut yogurt

Fermented foods: sauerkraut, kimchi, pickled ginger, fermented cucumbers, kombucha

Fiber: for a list of foods and their fiber content, go to the resources section at the end of the book. Fiber is what feeds your gut microbiome and makes you feel full. Fiber improves blood sugar control by binding sugar and releasing it slowly as you digest your food. It binds to cholesterol, lowering it, makes the bigger, fluffy, good kind of cholesterol, and lowers blood pressure and inflammation. Fiber also binds to toxic heavy metals, helping you to lower your accumulation of heavy metals.

Herbal teas

Low sugar content fruits: apricots, plums, apple, peach, pear, cherries, and berries, to name a few

Meats: fish, chicken, beef, lamb, organ meats, and so on. Preferably, eat grass-fed and hormone-free meats. Many of our farm-raised animals are fed corn that has been genetically modified or sprayed with glyphosate, which I have covered earlier in this chapter.

Most vegetables: asparagus, spinach, lettuce, broccoli, beets, cauliflower, carrots, celery, artichokes, garlic, onions, zucchini, squash, rhubarb, cucumbers, turnips, and watercress, among others

Olives and olive oil

Foods to Optimize Your Fiber Intake

Here is a suggestion of foods to eat to optimize your fiber intake to three cups of fruits, vegetables, and seeds a day:

2 fruits (such as 1 apple and 1 cup of berries)

1 tbsp. rice bran

1 tbsp. chia seeds

1 oz. dark chocolate

A more detailed listing of fiber in foods is provided in the resources section at the end of this book.

Eating at least 20–35 g of fiber each day is suggested by the American Dietetic Association.

Supplements

There are some specialized gut support products that help with gut lining healing repair, for when you have a leaky gut. Healing the gut lining reduces relapse or recurrence of digestive and immune system dysfunction. If you have a leaky gut that is mild, this process may take up to thirty days, a moderate occurrence will take up to sixty days, and severe leaky gut may take upwards of ninety days. You will need to eat in a way that helps balance your gut, as discussed above, and add in the extra supplements listed below.

Literature shows that these nutrients help repair and restore the gut lining. These supplements, which come in the form of a powder or a capsule, can be taken therapeutically from a few days up to three months, depending on the severity of gut impairment, the severity of symptoms, and your response to treatment.

Aloe leaf extract: This contains natural phytochemicals and powerful antioxidant properties that reduce intestinal inflammation, soothe the intestines, aid in intestinal wound healing, and have an anti-ulcer effect.

Gamma oryzanol: This is a mixture of plant sterols and ferulic acid esters from rice. It has been demonstrated to be a powerful antioxidant. It modulates and supports the enteric nervous system in its ability to activate intestinal motility and secrete digestive enzymes.[56]

L-Glutamine: This nonessential amino acid supports regeneration and repair of the intestinal lining. It has been shown to increase the number of cells in the small intestine and the number of villi on those cells, as well as the height of the villi.[57] Take 2,500 mg twice a day, either in capsule or powder form. This is the preferred fuel for the lining of the small intestine.

Marigold flower extract: This provides substrates for digestive enzyme production, reduces inflammation, and provides antibacterial activity. Its constituents include saponins, carotenoids, flavonoids, mucilage, bitter principle, phytosterols, polysaccharides, and resin.

Marshmallow extract: This has a high content of mucilage that can soothe and help heal compromised intestinal tissue. Endogenous hyaluronic acid is responsible for maintaining a degree of hydration of the skin and the lining of the intestine. Marshmallow root helps keep the levels of hyaluronic acid high because it inhibits hyaluronidase, an enzyme that is involved in the breakdown of hyaluronic acid, a necessary lubricant naturally produced by the body.

Quercetin: Take 500 mg twice a day with food and other flavonoids. It acts as a potent anti-inflammatory that helps restore the balance in the gut.

Slippery elm bark: This is very high in natural mucilage and is helpful in soothing inflamed intestinal cells. It reduces contact of inflammatory proteins with the intestinal mucosa, thereby enhancing recovery from intestinal barrier compromise and inflammation.

Biome medic: This is the only supplement brand on the market that shows a decrease in inflammation in the gut related to the absorption of Roundup. For the link to purchase it, see the resources section of the book.

This list of supplements is not exhaustive. Additional supplements will be required if *Candida*, parasites, or dysbiosis is found in the gut. This is why lab work and working with your doctor who is trained in this type of medicine (integrative medicine, holistic medicine, naturopathy, and/or functional medicine) is the best approach.

Lab Work

Microbiome

Your doctor can order a stool test to measure the diversity and robustness of your gut microbiome. You will be given a kit to take home. Collect your stool from the commode with a spatula and put it into the plastic test tube of the kit. The stool test also looks at inflammation levels in your gut, infections, yeast, parasites, and digestive enzymes. A healthy gut means a healthy brain!

Leaky Gut

There is also a blood test to check for inflammation in the gut caused by bacteria, foods, and/or stress. I like to use the company Cyrex Laboratories. The Cyrex blood test checks for zonulin, actinomycin, and LPS antibodies, the results of which provide your doctor with additional useful information. Cyrex Labs can also check for antibodies to specific foods, as well as aspects of the body, such as the joints, connective tissue, and even aspects of the brain cells. This lab can reveal the level of inflammation in the body, where it's coming from, and which part of the body it's affecting.

Zonulin

Our recent understanding of leaky gut and its relationship to autoimmune disease is based on the discovery of a protein called zonulin. Zonulin opens up the tight junctions of the intestinal wall and the junctions in the brain. When given to animal subjects, zonulin created immediate intestinal permeability. I mentioned celiac disease earlier in this chapter. For people with celiac disease, gluten triggers zonulin to open these junctions.

Actinomycin Antibodies

Actinomycin antibodies are another indication of intestinal destruction. Actinomycin is a complex of proteins that make up muscle fibers and contributes to muscular contractions. Actinomycin antibodies indicate gut damage that is severe enough to break through the cells, not just to open spaces between the cells. If actinomycin antibodies show up in your blood work, it usually means a longer period of time is needed to repair the gut lining, possibly six months or longer.

LPS Antibodies

LPS stands for *lipopolysaccharide*. This is a type of sugar molecule that is in the membrane of harmful bacteria, and it triggers inflammation. Immune cells in the mucosal lining of the gut do not interact with LPS unless the walls are breached due to the leaky gut. The presence of LPS antibodies can indicate gut flora abnormalities or an overgrowth of harmful bacteria in the digestive tract. When we see LPS antibodies in the bloodstream, we know it is causing inflammation throughout the body.

Cyrex Laboratories offer a test called Intestinal Antigenic Permeability Panel, which contains all three markers. This is a great place to start looking at brain healing. Lastly, Cyrex Labs does an excellent job at looking at the degree of gluten sensitivity you may have by looking at thirty-two different markers, as opposed to only the three to six done in regular lab testing.

Glyphosate

As I mentioned earlier in this chapter, Great Plains Lab is the only CLIA-certified lab that checks for glyphosate excretion by the body through the measurement of a single catch of urine.

6 COOLING BRAIN INFLAMMATION

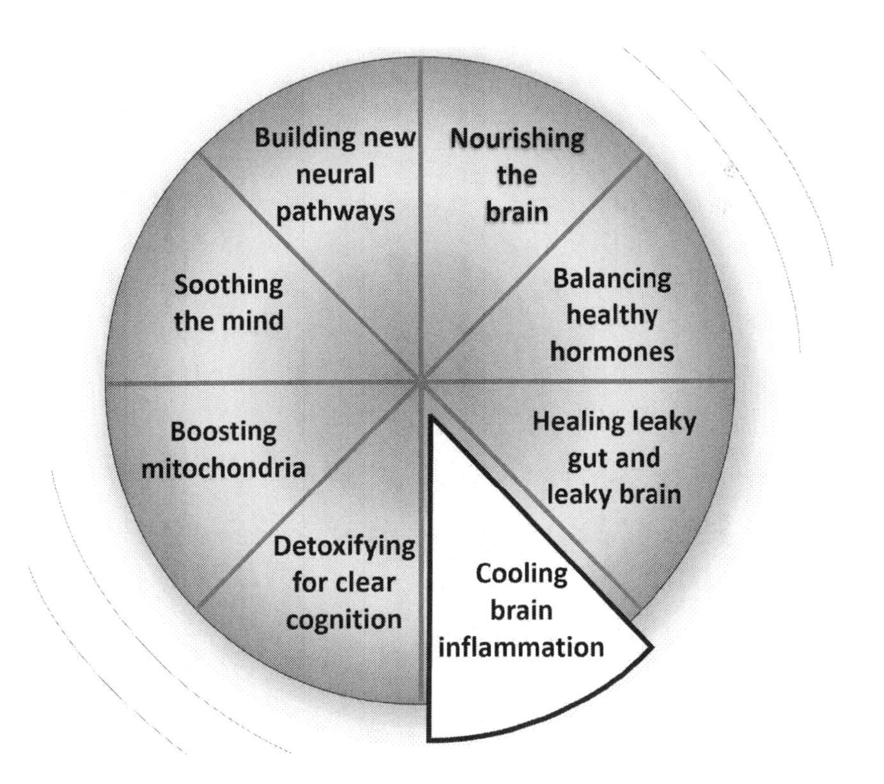

In the introduction, I outlined the major sections of the brain anatomically at a basic macroscopic level. In other words, if you were to hold a brain in your hands, you would see fissures, cracks, and smaller sections about the size of a tennis ball, of which at the most basic level there are three: the cerebrum (further divided into the left and right lobes), the cerebellum (which lies below the cerebrum), and the brain stem (which looks like a thick stem at the bottom of the brain).

If we now zoom in to look at the brain at a microscopic level, it consists of four major types of cells: neurons, oligodendrocytes, astrocytes, and microglia. The best-known are neurons, which we think of in colloquial terms as "nerve cells." Neurons oversee voluntary movement, emotions, and thoughts, and they also manage involuntary mechanisms, such as the rate of our heartbeat and our digestion.

As important as neurons are, however, they are a minority among the cells in our brains. The remaining three cell types support the neurons. The oligodendrocytes help make myelin, an insulating sheath crucial for increasing the speed of nerve transmission. You can think of the myelin as the rubber around an electrical cable. Myelin sheath destruction occurs in the neurodegenerative diseases such as multiple sclerosis and Parkinson's, both of which involve issues with muscle contraction.

The astrocytes are star-shaped glial cells in the brain and spinal cord. They provide the nutrient exchange that allows for biochemical support and ion balance. It's because of the astrocytes that ion waves, called intracellular calcium waves, pass over long distances in response to stimulation. So we could think of the astrocytes as being in charge of the electrical messaging system and bringing nutrients from the capillaries into the neurons of the brain.

This leaves us with the third cell type, the microglia, which comprise the brain's immune system, as mentioned earlier. The microglia sweep our brain looking for any infection they can clear.

Neuroglial Cells is a two-minute YouTube video showing our neuroanatomy at the cellular level.[58]

Inflammation results when your body detects problems like an infection, an irritation, toxins, or foreign molecules. White blood cells that kill infections mobilize chemicals called cytokines, which fight toxins, disease, and other foreign invaders. But sometimes the response is overzealous, which leads to diseases related to too much inflammation: autoimmune conditions, asthma, cancer, diabetes, cardiovascular disease, and others. In addition, the brain sometimes has a hard time turning off the inflammatory switch, which may lead to excessive or chronic inflammation in the brain itself.

Inflammation in the brain causes a cascade of damaging effects, such as these:

> Cells get triggered prematurely into a death cycle called *apoptosis*.
>
> Cellular enzymes become derailed.
>
> Neurotransmitters become ineffective.
>
> Receptor sites on cell membranes don't send signals well.
>
> Mental processing is slowed.

Various brain diseases are triggered by too much inflammation. These will be different for different people, but among them are autism, dementia, and depression. Since the Human Genome Project, which decoded the human genome, the scientific community unveiled a whole new view of how our genes affect our health. The study of *nutrigenomics* was born, which is a study of how our nutritional status affects our genetic expression.

Beth Ellen DiLullo, MS, RDN, LDN, states the following in an article posted on *Previmedica.com* (January 19, 2015), "Understanding MTHFR Genetic Mutation"[59]:

> *Current research in nutrigenomics indicates that some individuals, due to their unique genetic patterns and expression, do not produce adequate or effective MTHFR. The genetic variations in DNA sequencing are known as single nucleotide polymorphisms (SNPs). Ultimately MTHFR SNPs can cause hyper-homocysteinemia (especially if folate levels are low); affect nervous system, behavioral, and vascular health; contribute to birth defects, miscarriage, and preeclampsia; modulate cancer risk; and increase chronic disease risk.*
>
> *An estimated 50% of a population may have inherited one copy (heterozygous C/T) while up to 25% may have inherited two copies*

(homozygous T/T) ... individuals homozygous for C677T have at least a 50–60% reduction in MTHFR activity at body temperature (98.6°F/37°C).

Based on the current research, one can conclude that roughly 30 percent of the population does not detoxify chemicals and substances very well. They have genetic defects in their methylation pathways, which are pathways that allow for the breakdown of toxic substances, including alcohol and caffeine and other things such as pesticides, food coloring, and artificial flavorings.

Potential Causes of Inflammation

Here is a list of things that can cause inflammation in the brain:

A diet filled with foods that trigger inflammation (sugar, charcoaled meats, alcohol)

Common nutritional deficiencies (discussed above)

Direct or indirect physical trauma to the brain related to an injury in the neck, back, or sacrum

Food allergens

Imbalances in digestive function and the gut's immune system

Low-grade, hidden, or chronic infections

Sedentary lifestyle

Sleeping less than seven hours a night

Stress of all kinds: emotional, physical, and traumatic

Toxins such as mercury and pesticides

We have already elucidated dietary, gut, and toxin issues as causes of inflammation. Oral infections such as those involved in gum disease have been found to be seven times higher in those with Alzheimer's disease. Aside from the typical oral bacteria (specifically *Porphyromonas gingivalis*), other bacteria such as those from the gut microbiome (*Escherichia coli* and *Salmonella typhosa*) have been found causing disease through amyloid deposition. Other infections that have been associated with the progression of dementia are *Borrelia burgdorferi*, *Chlamydophila pneumoniae*, *Cytomegalovirus*, *Helicobacter pylori*, and herpes simplex virus type 1. Treating infections of the brain is beyond the scope of this book, but it is an important aspect of brain care that your physician can help you with.[60]

Emotional stress, physical trauma, and poor sleep will be addressed in the chapters to follow.

Trauma, the Vagus Nerve, and Brain Inflammation

Trauma can be caused by a physical blow to the head, an emotional "blow" to the heart, or an infectious onslaught that overwhelms our immune system. Such injuries can cause the primary network in our nervous system, called the central autonomic network, to gang up on our vagus nerve and inhibit it. The vagus nerve, which is also known as the tenth cranial nerve, can be thought of as a superhighway for nerves connecting our body to our brain. It is intimately involved in the autonomic nervous system, which coordinates our breathing rate; heartbeat; and internal water, nutrient, and gas balances. The vagus nerve is essentially playing a large role in our homeostasis, which is the tendency of a system—in this case our nervous system—to

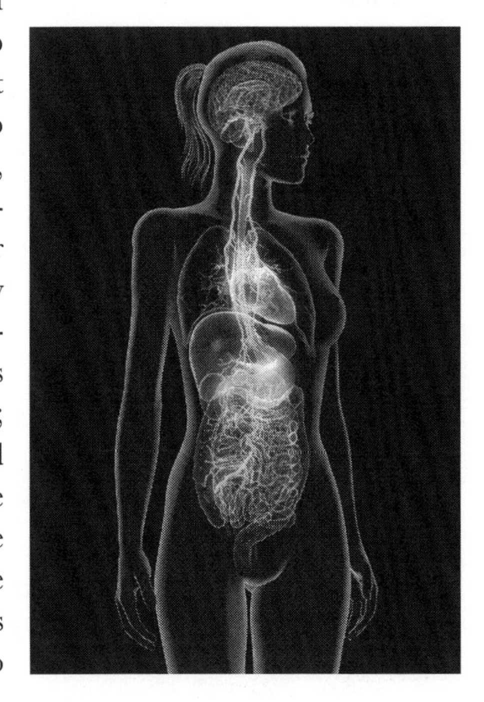

maintain an internal stability as a coordinated response of its parts to any situation or stimulus that tends to disturb our normal function.

The balancing act of the autonomic nervous system can be partitioned into two primary parts: the sympathetic nervous system and the parasympathetic nervous system. The sympathetic nervous system is the part of our nervous system that says "go, go, go." It acts like our accelerator, and when it is on, it gives us a sense of increased energy, with elevated blood pressure, mobilization of energy reserves, and increased heart rate. The parasympathetic nervous system, on the other hand, is the part of our nervous system that puts the brakes on and helps us to rest, digest our food, and relax.

The vagus nerve oversees 75 percent of our parasympathetic system. When the parasympathetic nervous system is stimulated, it decreases the heart rate and blood pressure, slows breathing, and increases the motility and blood flow of our digestive tract. It also promotes elimination from our bowel and bladder and aids in sexual arousal. When the vagus nerve gets inhibited, this causes dizziness, heart palpitations, a feeling as though your on-and-off stress switch is hyper reactive, indigestion, diarrhea and constipation. When the vagus nerve is inhibited we have more inflammation.[61] In fact, inflammation and white matter degeneration can persist for years after a single traumatic brain injury.

In 2011, researchers at the University of Amsterdam implanted vagus nerve stimulators into eight patients with severe rheumatoid arthritis (an autoimmune inflammatory condition that causes swollen, tender joints), and after forty-two days of having the vagus nerve stimulated for one to four minutes a day, most patients experienced a reduction in their symptoms and two of them had a complete remission.[62]

Stimulating the vagus nerve can also be helpful in depression. It's been noted in rat studies that the vagus nerve has an anti-inflammatory effect on the body, and if the loop connecting the brain to the organs by the vagus nerve is severed, then there is no anti-inflammatory effect. After a traumatic brain injury, the vagus nerve is often inhibited, resulting in more brain inflammation. In fact, brain inflammation and white matter degeneration can persist for years after a traumatic brain injury that harms the vagus nerve.

Traumatic brain injuries (TBIs) can damage the axons in the brain—that is, the nerve fibers that act like the arms and legs of our neurons by transmitting our neurological impulses from neuron to neuron. Because of a TBI, axons can undergo shearing, tearing, or stretching. When the axons are distorted in this way, the microtubules inside the neuron cells that deliver nutrients and chemical messages begin to shrivel and break down. As a result, a toxic inflammatory chemical called *glutamate* gets dumped into the space. In addition, the mitochondria, which produce energy packets called adenosine triphosphate (ATP) in each cell, get flooded in a soup of ions that makes it difficult for them to function.

Other physiological consequences may also occur. The cerebral blood flow can collapse, leading to a tremendous amount of oxidative stress, which impairs the stability of our DNA—our genes—in the most important organ of our body, our brain. The microglia, which are our brain's white blood cells, become aroused and hyperactive. The brain trauma creates more inflammation in the brain, and this inflammation can last for years. Symptoms can include headaches, dizziness, fainting, balance problems, exercise intolerance, forgetfulness, trouble concentrating, fatigue, and insomnia.

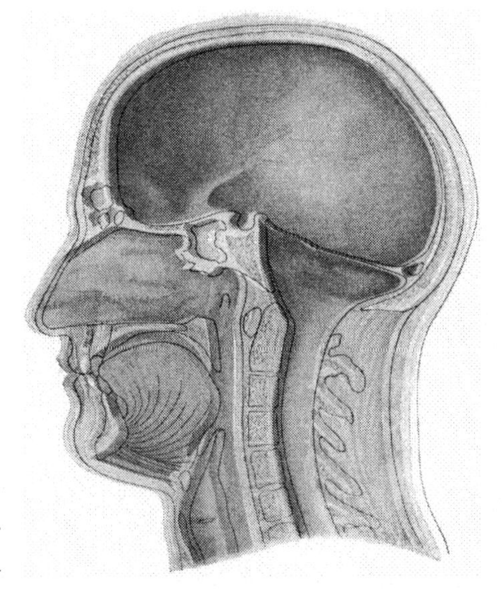

When I had my second and third brain injuries in 2018 from two car accidents (I was not driving the car in either of these), I didn't sustain any obvious outward injuries. I didn't have whiplash pain or a headache, but because of my previous injury when I fell off my bike at age fourteen, the tissues in my brain were less flexible the second and third times around. What I mean by *less flexible* is that the membranes that formed inside my brain were scarred from the old injury and were therefore less flexible and less resilient after the injury thirty-five years later. The membranes I'm alluding to are the *falx cerebri* (which is a very thick, double-layered fold of membrane that houses the major central vein in the brain) and the *falx cerebellli* (which is located at the back of the skull, near the base where the skull meets the neck—the cervical vertebrae). This part of the skull is where the cerebellum sits, hence the name *falx cerebelli*. As a result, my main symptom after these car accidents, in which I was rear-ended both times, was constipation. That may seem puzzling to many of you reading this. The result was constipation because the vagus nerve, passing through the lower part of my skull (specifically, the *jugular foramen*), had to pass through a restricted and tightened membrane. Since this area is so close to the neck muscles that hold the skull onto my cervical vertebrae, anything that created tension in my neck muscles, such as typing on the computer, sitting at a desk, or driving for long periods, would tend to lead to pressure on my vagus nerve, resulting in constipation and dizziness.

I learned to do stretching exercises for my vagus nerve and received cranial osteopathic manipulation (which you will learn about in the next chapter). I will review these exercises during our office visit together. The stretching resolved my constipation issue because it balanced my vagus nerve.

Let us return to the parasympathetic nervous system and to the benefits of relaxation with regard to your sympathetic nervous system, which is part of your stress response. Although we can't stop how we react to stress, we can help ourselves relax after the fact. Your relaxation response is wired into the part of your nervous system that you do have conscious control over—your parasympathetic nervous system. The nerve that controls this system is your vagus nerve. Every time you stimulate it, you set off the relaxation response.

The vagus nerve runs from the brain down through the body and into the diaphragm. This means that every time you take a deep breath in, you stimulate the vagus nerve and set off a cascade of positive effects in your body that improve your mental and physical health. In summary, some of the benefits of relaxation are these:

Enhanced neurogenesis, which helps you regenerate your entire body

Improved anti-inflammatory reactions

Improved heart rate variability

Cranial Osteopathic Manipulation

One powerful way to regain an inner sense of resiliency and optimize the functioning of the vagus nerve is by receiving a cranial osteopathic manipulation treatment by a skilled practitioner.

What is *cranial osteopathy*? *Cranium* means "head," and it is the skull that houses our brain. Cranial osteopathic manipulation is the therapeutic art of placing one's hands on the structure of the body in order to enhance its living anatomy. By *living*, I mean that our anatomy is not static—it is in motion at all times as a living and breathing organism. When we learn about the anatomy of the body, we are taught about it as though it were a static system—skeleton, muscles, tendons, ligaments, and organs—as though we were looking at a body on an operating table. However, our body is in constant motion, even when we are still and lying down.

Our Body Rhythms

Within this system are fluids flowing, muscular diaphragms contracting and relaxing, and our skeleton and muscles moving when we walk, sit, stand, jump, or squat.

Our body is also rhythmic:

Sixteen times a minute we breathe in, which makes our abdominal diaphragm move down several inches, pressing on our liver, spleen, and digestive organs before releasing and moving up.

Five liters a minute is the amount of blood being pumped through our circulatory system.

Sixty-five to a hundred times a minute is how often the ventricle chambers of our heart squeeze and pump oxygenated blood through our body system.

Eight to ten times a minute the cerebrospinal fluid in the brain and spinal cord swells and then recedes.

Dr. Sutherland Founds Cranial Osteopathy

The brain is a highly sensitive organ. That's why it's the only organ in our body that is protected by a helmet of bone, the skull, and bathed in a water balloon of protection called the *cerebrospinal fluid*. The cerebrospinal fluid flows back and forth like an ocean's tides, within the skull and alongside the spinal column inside the dural membrane, a protective sack connected to the bones. Our brain and spinal cord are literally floating inside our skull and spinal column inside the dural membrane. Our precious spinal cord is housed inside our cervical, thoracic, and lumbar spines. The dural membrane and fluid go all the way from the skull down the cervical, thoracic, and lumbar spines, ending in the lumbar spine.

One-fifth of the body's blood supply is dedicated to the brain and the cerebrospinal fluid. Since the brain houses fluids that flow within membranes and down the spinal cord, there is a subtle motion that can be palpated and enhanced for maximum benefit of the body. The practice of cranial osteopathy was founded by an osteopathic physician, William Garner Sutherland, DO (1873–1954). Dr. Sutherland discovered, developed, and taught cranial osteopathy in the early to mid-1900s. He was the first to perceive a subtle palpable movement with the bones of the cranium.

He went on to discover the continuity of this rhythmic fluid movement throughout all tissues of the body. Just as the lungs breathe and the heart beats with a rhythmic alternating motion of expansion and contraction, the central nervous system has its own involuntary rhythmic motion. Dr. Sutherland called this inherent activity the *primary respiratory mechanism*, because it seemed to have a respiratory-like motion, with "inhalation" and "exhalation" phases. Dr. Sutherland viewed life as pulsating contractions and expansions that he called the "breath of life."

A Skilled Osteopathic Physician

The hands of a skilled osteopathic physician connect directly with this primary respiratory mechanism to initiate a therapeutic response. Primary respiration is the guiding principle; it is the inherent intelligence within. This primary respiratory motion actually expresses itself through every cell of the body, influencing all body functions. Physicians trained in cranial osteopathy can place their hands on any part of a person to perceive and influence this important mechanism.

The brain is covered by twenty-two skull bones. Connected to these skull bones are three membranes (or *meninges*): the dura mater, arachnoid mater, and pia mater. Floating between these membranes is the brain's cerebrospinal fluid. The cerebrospinal fluid courses down the entire spinal column from the brain and provides 80 percent of the nourishment to the spinal nerves. This quote is from the *Encyclopedia of Surgery*:

> [Cerebrospinal fluid] *contains glucose, electrolytes, amino acids, and other small molecules found in plasma, but has very little protein and few cells. Cerebrospinal fluid protects the central nervous system from injury, cushions it from the surrounding bone structure, provides it with nutrients, and removes waste products by returning them to the blood.*[63]

The skull bones are connected by these deep brain structures that can be palpated by an osteopathic doctor with skilled, gentle, light touch while the patient lies on a treatment table for about thirty minutes. A healthy craniosacral system pulsates at a rate of six to fifteen times a minute, noticeable by a subtle expansion of the cranial bones as the cerebrospinal fluid is being made, as well as a subtle contraction, or coming together, of the joints of the skull with the circulation of cerebrospinal fluid around the spine. These subtle motions of the bones in the skull have been objectively measured; they are called the Traube-Hering-Mayer oscillations. Through the intelligent application of focused and sensitive touch, the sutures, which move 0.01 mm, can be decompressed and the flow of cerebrospinal flow enhanced.

Other deep brain structures such as the vagus nerve allow the parasympathetic nervous system to help you relax. When the cranial rhythm is optimized, many people experience a deep feeling of calm and connectedness. There is a resynchronization of the health in your body.

Various Conditions Are Treated

The following conditions are commonly treated with cranial osteopathic manipulation:

Allergies and sinus congestion

Asthma

Cerebral palsy

Chronic infections, including ear infections

Chronic infectious disease

Colic

Delayed childhood development

Digestive disorders and upset

Dyslexia

Genitourinary problems

Headaches

Insomnia

Joint pain syndromes

Learning disorder

Low back pain

Neurological syndromes

Pediatric problems

Rheumatic problems

Sciatica

Seizure disorders

Spinal cord injury

Sucking difficulty in babies

Temporomandibular joint dysfunction

Trauma of the body, head, or neck

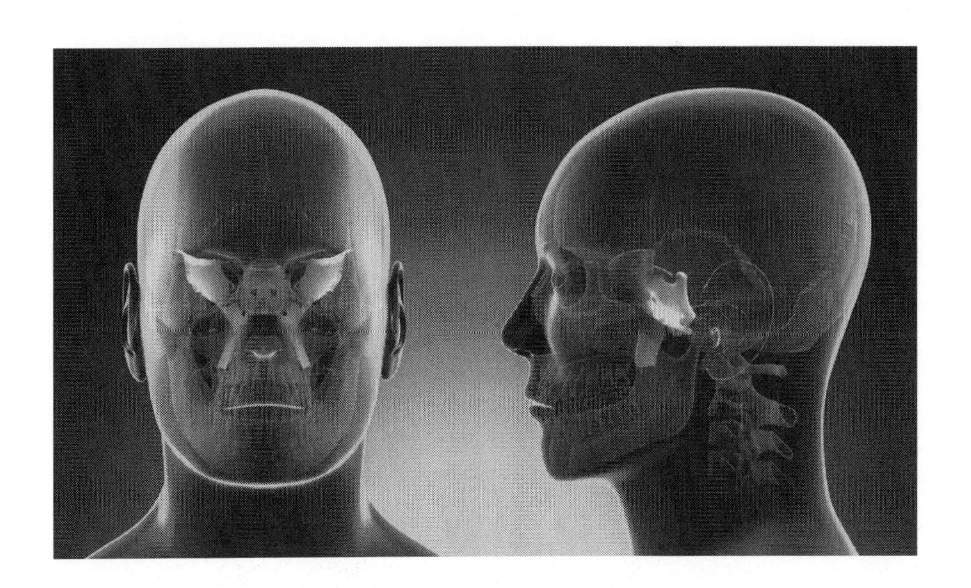

Blows to the Skull

In life we are prone to injuring or bruising our brain by falling and hitting our head, for example, when we fall off a bicycle, a ladder, or a skateboard, or when we ski. Such injuries can be quite frequent in sports such as football, ice hockey, and martial arts.

One of the most critical bones in the skull is the sphenoid bone. This bone houses part of the eyes by forming the back of the orbits in the skull. The back end of the sphenoid bone (called the *sella turcica*, Latin for "Turkish chair") houses the hypothalamus and pituitary, two of the most important endocrine organs in the body. The hypothalamus and pituitary produce key stimulating hormones (discussed in chapter 4, "Balancing Healthy Hormones") that direct the thyroid, adrenal, testes, and ovaries. This bone also plays a role in sinus function and the nerves that help with vision and eye movement. This bone looks like a bird with outstretched wings perched right behind the top of your nose, between the eyes. The tips of the wings of the bird touch the outer part of the eyes.

Blows to the face—such as a soccer ball smashing the head, or the side of the head hitting the side window of a car—can distort the sphenoid bone, especially if the blow connects with the side of the head or the back of head. Because the sphenoid bone houses the pituitary gland, hormonal issues can ensue. A blow to the cheekbones or temporal bone around the ear can compromise hearing and balance and cause dizziness. According to Dr. Maud Nerman, DO, author of *Healing Pain and Injury*, "Sphenoid distortion can thereby affect hormones, causing emotional chaos, poor healing, fatigue, and immune issues. There can be visual, sinus, and pain problems." Approximately 47 percent of all brain injuries affect the functioning of the pituitary gland.

A trained osteopath can evaluate the position of the bones of the skull. The sutures between the skull bones can be compressed, causing distortions and strain patterns on the membranes. Not only can the bones and membranes of the skull be assessed and their healthy movement optimized, but the inner part of the brain, the *parenchyma*, can undergo a relaxation from the increase in fluid flow. The central autonomic system governs our immunity, as well as certain areas such as the *locus coeruleus* (which produces the highest amount of norepinephrine or stress hormone in our bodies) and the amygdala. As I explain earlier in this chapter, the vagus nerve passes through a hole in the skull called the jugular foramen. The jugular vein also passes through this hole, just behind the ear at the base of the skull. If we fall on the side of our head, we can compress the jugular foramen. An osteopath can open up and balance this area. In fact, modern medicine recognizes the profound importance of the vagal nerve and has created vagal nerve stimulators, which are little mechanical devices that are surgically placed just under the skin near the vagal nerve output in those with ongoing seizures. We are noticing that the vagal nerve stimulators not only reduce inflammation but also reduce seizures.

Another benefit to receiving a cranial osteopathic manipulative treatment is that it helps with the toxin removal from the brain through the glymphatic system. Until recently, it was thought that the brain had no lymphatic system. Anatomists and scientists are now discovering that indeed it does—it's called the *glymphatic system*. This system allows for drainage of some nasty things:

Neurotoxins, such as heavy metals, particles of infectious organisms, pesticides, and chemicals

Proteins such as tau protein and amyloid beta protein, both of which are found to be built up in Alzheimer's disease

The result is increased health for the brain! When you receive cranial osteopathic manipulation, you are essentially getting a brain massage. Getting your brain massaged feels like you just returned from a two-week vacation.

Cranial osteopathic manipulation is one of my favorite forms of therapy. Recently, a patient received biweekly sessions for one month and for the first time in over ten years was able to sleep through the night, and her full-body numbness is going away.

I look forward to giving you a session to re-engage you with your inner health force.

The Basic Plan to Reduce Inflammation

Below is an outline of the steps to take to reduce inflammation in your body generally and your brain in particular:

Add anti-inflammatory spices such as turmeric, ginger, and rosemary to your diet.

Develop love, community, and connection.

Eat real, whole, hormone-free and pesticide-free foods.

Eliminate hidden food allergies.

Exercise regularly (see the section "The Benefits of Exercising" in chapter 8).

Get a cranial osteopathic treatment.

Get adequate sleep.

Heal emotional trauma (see chapter 9, "Soothing Your Mind").

Take helpful supplements and herbs

Supplement with Molecular Hydrogen

Molecular hydrogen (H_2) is a new supplement that may be one of the most basic and potentially beneficial therapies in existence for reducing inflammation in the central nervous system. Therapeutic application of H_2 dates back to the 1940s, when it was used for the prevention of decompression sickness in divers. The antioxidant principles and other biological effects broadly translate to numerous health benefits; 450 publications reflect over 170 different human and animal disease models.

In 2007, research findings published in *Nature Medicine* showed that inhaled H_2 gas, as well as H_2 dissolved in a liquid cellular nutrient solution, substantially decreased damage to the brain associated with *ischemia-reperfusion injury*, which is tissue damage caused when the blood supply returns to the tissue after a period of ischemia, or lack of oxygen. It does this by reducing the amount of hydroxyl radical (•OH) generated in the cytoplasm and in the nucleus of the cell. H_2 readily passes through cell membranes and the blood-brain barrier, as well as into all cellular compartments and biological tissues. Molecular H_2 has been studied as a therapy for numerous central nervous system diseases because of its antioxidant and anti-inflammatory properties.

Animal studies have shown that consumption of H_2-rich water reduced the loss of neurons in an animal model of Parkinson's disease.[64] Preclinical animal models suggest that treatment with H_2 may improve cognition and memory in those with Alzheimer's disease, as well as improve brain function under stress and aging.[65] In fact, in a double-blind, placebo-controlled crossover study, consumption of 600 ml of H_2-rich water (the equivalent of two and a half glasses) daily for four weeks was shown to significantly decrease psychological distress and sympathetic nerve activity in human volunteers at rest.[66]

Lab Work

With your doctor's help you can have lab work done to measure your inflammatory markers and determine the possible causes of inflammation that could be affecting your brain.

Almost all standard labs can order the test for high-sensitivity C-reactive protein (hs-CRP) in the blood, which can be a helpful way to track inflammation in your body. I like to see a level less than 0.3 mg/dl. Slightly elevated levels of 2–3 mg/dl indicate low-grade inflammation in the body, from infection, food allergies, or toxins, suggesting that further attention to lower inflammation as outlined here is wise. Nowadays, there are even more specific labs that measure a broader array of inflammatory markers, including the ones found in brain inflammation and dementia. When inflammation rises, the enzyme nitric oxide is often lowered. Nitric oxide is crucial for vasodilation and our circulation. I offer a spit test for nitric oxide levels as part of the lab work during your medical office visit.

7 DETOXIFYING FOR COGNITIVE CLARITY

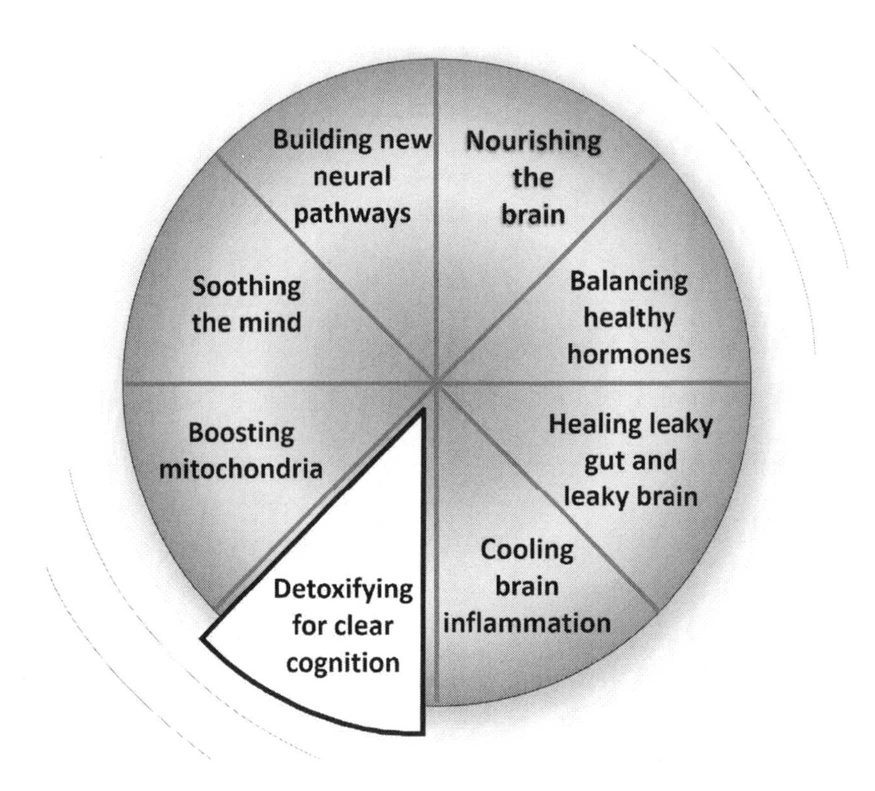

Almost all of us know someone who has or has had cancer. A cancer diagnosis is one that no one wants to get: the treatment can be brutal, expensive, and taxing on ourselves and our loved ones, and it can lead to our life ending earlier than desired. There have been breakthroughs in cancer therapy, but the best therapy is not to get it in the first place. Although toxins have never been directly implicated as causes of cancer, I once spoke with an oncologist at a medical conference who confided to me that "80 percent of cancer is caused by environmental toxins. We just don't go around talking about it as a medical community, because there's nothing you can do about it."

This made sense to me. So often, many people who are not smokers or drinkers and who have a relatively healthy lifestyle with a good diet, exercise, and loving relationships develop cancer. Why do these people get cancer? The answer to this question lies in the lives and deaths of some of our furry friends. Animals in the wild, as well as our domesticated buddies, don't have "bad" self-imposed behaviors and toxic lifestyles, such as eating too much sugar, drinking alcohol, and smoking. And yet animals are getting cancer at alarmingly high rates. Bladder cancer rates among dogs, whales, sea life, and even birds are on the increase.

Living a low-toxin lifestyle and doing lab work to make sure your body is detoxifying well can be one of the best things you can do to prevent cancer.

Unfortunately, we live in a sea of toxins. Since the late 1800s, more than 80,000 new chemicals have been introduced into our environment. Only about 6 percent of them have been tested for their long-term effects on human health, and those that have been tested do not bode well for what the rest of them are doing to our bodies and our brains. Toxins are everywhere, from household cleaners to plastics in kitchenware. They are in our water and air supply, in our cosmetics, and even in our food. These toxins are responsible for the epidemic of disease we see in the twenty-first century.

Four Steps to Living Healthfully

We need to take four steps to handle living in a toxic world:

Identify toxins in your home environment, in cleaning products, scented candles, new furniture, cookware, and personal care products such as shampoos and cosmetics.

Identify toxins in your body through the lab work that I describe later in this chapter.

Get rid of toxins by enhancing the detoxification system in your own body.

Avoid further toxin exposure by living a clean lifestyle.

This excerpt is from the Environmental Working Group's website (ewg.org):

> *Hundreds of everyday products are made with highly toxic fluorinated chemicals called PFAS. They build up in our bodies and never break down in the environment. Very small doses of PFAS have been linked to cancer, reproductive and immune system harm, and other diseases.*
>
> *For decades, chemical companies covered up evidence of PFAS' health hazards. Today nearly all Americans, including newborn babies, have PFAS in their blood, and up to 110 million people may be drinking PFAS-tainted water.*
>
> ...
>
> *In 1946 DuPont introduced nonstick cookware coated with Teflon. Today the family of fluorinated chemicals that sprang from Teflon includes thousands of nonstick, stain-repellent, and waterproof compounds called PFAS, short for per- and poly-fluoroalkyl substances.*
>
> *PFAS are used in a staggering array of consumer products and commercial applications. Decades of heavy use have resulted in contamination of water, soil, and blood of people and animals in the farthest corners of the world. PFAS are incredibly persistent, never breaking down in the environment and remaining in our bodies for years.*[67]

Heavy Metal Toxicity: Mercury

The phrase "mad as a hatter" (alluded to in the Mad Hatter character in *Alice in Wonderland*) is what we think of when we think of mercury poisoning. Mercurous nitrate was once used in curing felt to make top hats, and prolonged exposure to mercury vapors caused mercury poisoning. Mercury is the second most neurotoxic chemical on the planet. It viciously attacks the nervous system, brain, and kidneys.

Sources of Mercury

The three primary sources of mercury are (1) silver dental fillings, also known as amalgams, which are 50 percent mercury; (2) coal-soaked air that contaminates our environment; and (3) most large ocean fish—such as tuna, mahi-mahi, and swordfish—which bio-magnify the mercury they consume in smaller fish. We must minimize the sources of mercury toxicity we consume and help our bodies detoxify the rest by supporting our detoxification systems.

What Does Mercury Actually Do in the Body?

Mercury toxicity disrupts the function of our enzymes. When they don't work, the transport of minerals into our cells is diminished. This leads to an overproduction of reactive oxygen species and impaired ATP production by the mitochondria. ATP is what energizes every reaction in the body, so the end result is that we feel tired.

Symptoms of mercury toxicity include these:

- ADD in children and staring spells
- Blurred vision
- Headaches
- Insomnia
- Irritability
- Neuropathy, showing up as unusual sensations or unsteady gait
- Personality changes
- Slowed mental response
- Tremors
- Weakness and fatigue

Mercury also interferes with how our hormones function. It does this by inhibiting methylation, which is a biochemical process that affects the production of many hormones and neurotransmitters. One of the particular enzymes that mercury blocks is the methionine synthase enzyme. We need this enzyme in order to recycle and regenerate our hormones and balance our brain chemistry.

Mercury concentrates in glands, including the thyroid and pituitary glands, where it blocks the enzyme that converts inactive thyroid hormone to active thyroid hormone. When your thyroid is blocked, you may feel tired, lethargic, cold, and constipated.

Mercury also depletes glutathione, which is a protective antioxidant in the brain and liver, and it blocks the enzyme that regenerates glutathione. Mercury damages the tight junctions in the intestinal wall, which can lead to leaky gut and leaky blood-brain barrier. Mercury activates the phospholipase enzymes that break down membranes. Cell membranes can only withstand so much damage, but too much can cause them to die.

In blood vessels, mercury causes vascular endothelial dysfunction, which causes reduced blood flow to the brain and other organs. There is a lab test for matrix metalloproteinase-9 (MMP-9) activity, a blood draw that can be done to see if this process is going on in your body.

As you can see, mercury can wreak havoc on your biochemistry and hormones. Many of the symptoms of mercury toxicity come from how mercury affects the brain. In the brain, mercury causes microglial activation—that's an immune response—as well as neuro-inflammation in general. Mercury alters the redox balance within cells, pushing it toward oxidation rather than reduction, which is undesirable. This redox balance is important because it determines the activity of many brain enzymes, meaning that with mercury, your brain is always on, and it doesn't get enough rest. One key brain neurotransmitter that helps us naturally calm down is gamma-aminobutyric acid (GABA). I call it our natural "chill" molecule. It's also what Ativan, Valium, or a nice glass of wine raises in your body to help calm you down. Mercury disrupts GABA in the brain in several ways. It blocks glutamic acid decarboxylase, the enzyme that synthesizes GABA. Mercury also blocks certain GABA receptors and causes a selective loss of Purkinje neurons in the brain, the neurons that produce GABA.

Mercury is a neurotoxin. It literally poisons your brain cells to death. It also blocks many metabolic pathways, including those related to building new hemoglobin molecules (oxygen-carrying molecules inside your red blood cells). This seems to be linked to the neurotoxin and neurobehavioral effects of the chemical. I have highlighted mercury as one of the heavy metals most toxic to our brain, but there are others, and they have a synergistic toxic effect. Other heavy metals to be aware of are arsenic, cadmium, lead, and aluminum, which the Agency for Toxic Substances and Disease Registry lists as among the top five of the 275 most hazardous substances in the environment.

For women, cosmetics can be a source of heavy metal toxicity. Use clean products on your skin. If you wear makeup, consult the Environmental Working Group's Skin-Deep Guide before purchasing cosmetics.[68] They have a database that rates the toxicity levels of thousands of different products. This is especially important for lipstick, a common source of lead.[69]

Lab Work for Toxic Heavy Metals

Lab work can look for toxic heavy metals in the body, such as mercury, lead, cadmium, and arsenic. Blood lead and mercury levels will only show what you have been carrying in your body for the past 120 days. Heavy metals are stored long term in your bones and organs and can stay there for sixty years! Therefore, the most accurate way to assess chronic body burden is to do a provoked urine test using chelating agents DMPS, DMSA, or CaEDTA. These chelating agents are obtained with a doctor's prescription. These medications bind to the metals in your body and carry them out through your stool and urine. If you have silver amalgam fillings in your teeth, it may be advisable to have them removed and replaced with porcelain or all gold before you detox from heavy metals. If you decide to do this, make sure that your dentist is trained in oral toxicology. You can contact the International Academy of Oral Medicine and Toxicology to find a dentist in your area who is trained in this way.[70]

Other Toxic Agents That Poison Us

Heavy metals aren't the only chemicals we are exposed to that create toxicity for us. Other such chemicals that affect us are these:

Pesticides

Phthalates in plastic water bottles

Numerous other environmental toxins and petrochemicals

Volatile organic compounds (VOCs)

Consider the example of Parkinson's, which has been irrefutably linked to toxic exposure. Some forms of depression, dementia, and Alzheimer's have been linked to toxic exposure as well. Some people are more exposed to toxins if they live near agricultural farms, drink or cook with water that has been exposed to toxins, live near highways, and have genes that don't break down toxins very well.

The good news is that despite the large burden of toxins in our system today, your body has the ability to detoxify from even some of the most insidious chemical agents.

In fact, there is one chemical that does most of this work for us. It is known as the master detoxifier of your body, the "mother of all antioxidants," and the maestro of the immune system. It is called *glutathione*.

Glutathione: The Master Detoxifier

Glutathione is one of the most powerful antioxidants in our body. It is made from three major components: the amino acids glutamate, glycine, and cysteine. Glutathione is stored in the liver, kidneys, lungs, and small intestine. As one of the body's most powerful antioxidants, it helps recycle other antioxidants such as vitamin C and vitamin E. Glutathione binds to fat-soluble toxins and makes them water-soluble, so they can be excreted. Glutathione binds to heavy metals, helping escort them out of our bodies. It regulates cellular replication. Lastly, it boosts our immune system by increasing regulation of the function of natural killer cells.

When would we need more glutathione in our body? We may need more glutathione if there is an imbalance between how much we make and how much is needed. In other words, if the demand outweighs the supply.

Things that reduce our supply of glutathione are these:

Acetone (for example, from manicures and pedicures)

Alcohol (more than one glass of wine a day for a woman or two glasses of wine a day for a man)

Chlorine in the water

Electromagnetic smog

Environmental toxins (such as highway pollution, herbicides, and pesticides)

Fire retardant on furniture

Food dyes

Formaldehydes (for instance, in household furnishings)

Gasoline fumes

Heavy metals (dental amalgams and large fish are the main sources)

Indoor cleaning materials

Lifestyle factors (such as excessive caffeine and alcohol)

Nitrates (high in salami, hot dogs, cured meats)

Non-stick cookware

Oxidative stress (from intense physical exercise, infection, or emotional stress)

Pesticides
Plastics
Pollutants
Tylenol
UV radiation
X-rays

After age thirty, our production of glutathione naturally starts decreasing.[71]

This is also why diseases such as cancer, arthritis, and heart disease tend to happen later in life, when part of our antioxidant system is less active.

Lab Work for Glutathione

The problem with glutathione testing is that glutathione oxidizes very rapidly, so when a blood level is to be checked, that blood sample has to be put on ice immediately, otherwise it reduces to an oxidized form and the reading is inaccurate. Indirect testing is helpful and sometimes better because of this issue. A common blood test that every lab at a hospital or outpatient clinic can do is called gamma-glutamyl transferase (GGT). GGT enzyme is made in the liver and increases with organophosphate toxicity, as well as with too much alcohol. If the GGT is increased, this indicates a need for more glutathione.

Another test that can be done is a urine organic amino acids test. If N-acetyl cysteine (NAC) levels are low on this test or the 2-OH butyric acid is high, this indicates a need for glutathione. Lastly, a new test called *DNA oxidative damage*, a urine test, looks at the oxidative stress on DNA. This test measures our antioxidant reserves. If we have enough reserves to meet the level of oxidant stress in our lives, then our DNA oxidative damage will be normal. If our oxidative stress exceeds our antioxidant levels, then our DNA oxidative damage will be elevated. This is an effective way to see if you are taking enough antioxidants to buffer the effects of the stressors your body is under. Remember that antioxidant stress is something we don't actually feel in our body, until the dreaded disease occurs, and by then it is much harder to reverse, as in the case of heart disease, arthritis, and cancer, for example.

Glutathione Depletion

What can you do if your glutathione is depleted?

Get an IV of glutathione through one of the veins in your arm. A nurse at your doctor's office may be able to perform this. Glutathione IVs have been used for neurological illnesses such as ALS, dementia, Parkinson's, and MS. Studies show that although a glutathione IV reduces symptoms by 42 percent, all the symptoms come back about two weeks after the IVs stop. IVs are time-consuming and expensive, so this can be challenging, although worth it for a person with a severe neurological condition such as the ones mentioned above.

Most oral glutathione does not cross the blood-brain barrier and is poorly absorbed.

Fortunately, there is a new form, which can be obtained at the medical offices that carry the brand Researched Nutritionals. It is liposomal, meaning it crosses the blood-brain barrier. Studies done on this brand in particular show that within two weeks of taking it, the natural killer cell activity in the body increases by 400 percent, and in two weeks lipid peroxidation goes down 25 percent. This form is GMO free and heat stable.

Basic Plan for Detoxification

Most of us think that a healthy lifestyle means a good diet and exercise, but now that you have learned about toxins and their damaging effects to our bodies, I propose that detoxification is just as important as a good diet and exercise, and that we should incorporate detoxification into our regime once or twice a year. Detoxification is a process that can take as little as four days, ten days, or as long as twenty-one days. Spring and summer are the best seasons to detoxify, as these are the ones that encourage our body to shed the old and the time when we have more energy. Winter is not a good time to detoxify, as our body is encouraged to hold on to our fat as the nights get longer, and the body naturally shifts into more of a hibernation mode.

The detoxification process has several components (about which I will go into more detail below):

Living a clean lifestyle

Supplements for enhancing detoxification

Diet

Working with your doctor to enhance detoxification

Preparing for detoxification

Sauna or hyperthermia therapy

Living a Clean Lifestyle

A critical part of regenerating your brain is reducing your toxic exposure by living a clean and green lifestyle. Eliminating as many toxins from your environment as possible is as essential as enhancing your detoxification.

This is from the website of the Environmental Working Group (EWG):

> *The US Centers for Disease Control and Prevention found detectable levels of BPA in 93 percent of samples taken in 2003–04 from people six years and older. In 2009, tests commissioned by EWG were the first to find BPA in the umbilical cords of nine out of ten infants sampled. BPA is one of twenty-three biologically disruptive chemicals being investigated by the Halifax Project, an international collaboration of scientists and doctors who are studying the connection between chemical exposures and cancer.*[72]

BPA plastic is used in our water bottles, our plastic food storage containers, the plastic wrap around our meat in the grocery store, and in the lining of cans such as coffee bean cans, canned soups, and even beer kegs.

Researchers from Texas A&M University found that mice ingesting BPA at levels commonly found in the American diet triggered inflammatory bowel symptoms commonly seen in ulcerative colitis. Inflammatory bowel disease (IBD) also includes issues like Crohn's disease symptoms.

According to Clint Allred, MD, "Because humans are frequently exposed to BPA through consumption of canned foods and the use of polycarbonate plastic containers, it's important to find out just what effects BPA exposure may have on IBD. To this end, we investigated the effects of BPA exposure in a pre-clinical model using mice with IBD."

In collaboration with the laboratory group of Arul Jayaraman, PhD, from the chemical engineering department at Texas A&M, Dr. Allred and his research team investigated the ability of BPA to exacerbate colonic inflammation and alter microbiota metabolites derived from aromatic amino acids in an acute dextran sulfate sodium-induced colitis model.

"We assessed body weight and fecal consistency in addition to inflammation, injury and nodularity of the colon," Dr. Allred explained. "We also analyzed changes in microbiota metabolite levels derived from aromatic amino acids reflecting changes in the gut microbiome."

Exposure to BPA also increased the levels of several compounds that drive inflammation in the colon, Allred said.

"Scat from animals exposed to BPA had reduced levels of compounds produced by gut bacteria from the breakdown of protein, including tryptophan and 5-hydroxy indole 3-acetic acid," he said. "These compounds are related to serotonin production and breakdown, and their reduction has been linked with IBD."

Allred said comprehensive study results showed BPA exposure increased mortality and worsened disease symptoms when compared to untreated groups.[73]

Vitamin D drain

A study published in September 2016 in the Endocrine Society's *Journal of Clinical Endocrinology & Metabolism* found that people who were exposed to larger amounts of phthalates were more likely to have low levels of vitamin D in the bloodstream than the participants who were exposed to smaller amounts of the hormone-disrupting chemicals. There also was an association between exposure to higher levels of BPA and reduced vitamin D levels in women, although the relationship was not statistically significant in men. Vitamin D deficiency is linked to all sorts of health problems, including things like weight gain, cancer, insomnia, arthritis, heart disease, MS, and other ills.[74]

Researchers say hormone disruptors could mess with the active form of vitamin D in the body in a similar way that they disrupt normal reproductive and thyroid function.

Obesity breeder

In 2013, Kaiser Foundation Research Institute scientists who closely evaluated the urine BPA levels in 1,326 school-aged children from Shanghai linked BPA to obesity. They found that girls who had a higher urine BPA level were twice as likely to be obese as the average of the other children.[75]

Erratic heartbeats

In 2011, scientists published a study that revealed more specifics about BPA's link to heart disease. The *PLOS One* article found BPA actually changed the natural heartbeat signaling in female rats. This led to arrhythmia, an erratic beating that sometimes causes sudden cardiac death.[76]

BPA is not the only problem. Instead of using bisphenol A, manufacturers are now using bisphenol S (BPS) and other chemicals. Yet recent studies are proving that this new approach is just as bad (if not worse) than using BPA. In fact, recent reports claim that more than

80 percent of Americans have detectable levels of BPS in their urine. And according to a 2013 study out of the University of Texas Medical Branch at Galveston, even less than one part per trillion of intracellular BPS can disrupt a cell's normal functioning, which could potentially lead to metabolic disorders such as diabetes, obesity, asthma, birth defects, and even cancer.[77]

It seems that the problem is everywhere. In 2011 the journal *Environmental Health Perspectives* published a very shocking study in which scientists evaluated 455 plastic products that were purchased from Albertsons, H-E-B, Randall's, Target, Walmart, Trader Joe's, and Whole Foods. The study's specific purpose was to determine whether or not BPA-free products release chemicals having estrogenic activity (EA), which has been linked to serious health effects at extremely low *nanomolar* (barely detectible) levels. The researchers reported, "Almost all commercially available plastic products we sampled—independent of the type of resin, product, or retail source—leached chemicals having reliably detectable EA, including those advertised as BPA free. In some cases, BPA-free products released chemicals having more EA than did BPA-containing products."[78]

Tips for avoiding BPA and BPS

Here are some tips for avoiding BPA and BPS:

Buy organic food as much as possible.

Switch from using plastic containers (especially Tupperware and plastic water bottles) to glass or stainless steel whenever possible.

Avoid storing food in plastic, especially plastics #3, #6, and #7. The Institute of Functional Medicine states this:

#3 Vinyl or PVC. Most commercial cling wrap, plastic bottles used for olive and cooking oil, some water bottles. The risks are suspected hormone disruptors and carcinogens.

#6 PS (polystyrene). Disposable plastic cups and bowls, most opaque plastic cutlery. The risks are carcinogens and suspected hormone disruptors.

#7 Other (usually polycarbonate [PC]). Most clear plastic baby bottles, five-gallon water jugs, clear plastic sippy cups, some clear plastic cutlery, and Nalgene drink bottles. The risks are that many contain BPA, which is known to be an endocrine disruptor.

One of the best ways to detoxify from plastic is by sweating it out. According to an article published in the National Institutes of Health (NIH), when the phthalate levels were measured in the blood, urine, and sweat of 20 individuals, the metabolite of plastic was found in the sweat but not in the blood, and was twice as high as in urine. This suggests two things: plastics bioaccumulate in our bodies, and sweating them out is the only scientifically proven method of elimination that we know of to date. A weekly sauna regime is an excellent way to do this, which I will further elucidate in this chapter.[79]

Supplements for Enhancing Detoxification

The most important factor for our detoxification system is keeping our glutathione levels up. As I have explained, glutathione is the main detoxifier in the body. Our body needs to regenerate itself all the time. That is why we need to keep the sulfation and methylation trains running smoothly. Our brains and health depend on them.

Although my favorite glutathione supplement is liposomal glutathione, there are other routes and ways to get toxins out of the body. These pathways require many helpers for our detox system to function day in and day out: vitamins, minerals, amino acids, special nutrients, and a whole range of phytonutrients.

The main nutrients helpful in boosting glutathione include all the methylation nutrients from cruciferous vegetables (such as broccoli and cauliflower), B12, folic acid, zinc, and selenium, all of which are part of your basic supplements package in the eight-week Regenerate Your Brain Program that I deliver through my offices.

Additional supplements include these:

N-acetylcysteine (NAC), 500 mg twice a day. This is a special amino acid that dramatically increases glutathione. It is even used in the emergency room to treat liver failure from Tylenol overdose.

Buffered ascorbic acid (vitamin C), 1000 mg twice a day in addition to what is in your most basic multivitamin.

Milk thistle (silymarin), 140 mg twice a day of standardized extract. This herb has long been used in liver disease and helps boost glutathione levels.

The Detox Diet

Although I have already discussed a diet that is healthy for the brain overall and another diet that is more restrictive and specific to leaky gut, there is also a type of diet that is specially adapted for detoxification. Certain foods are particularly potent supporters of liver detoxification. I have recommended one such class before—they are called cruciferous vegetables. This class includes cabbage, broccoli, collards, kale, brussels sprouts, Chinese cabbage, bok choy, arugula, radishes, wasabi, watercress, kohlrabi, mustard greens, rutabaga, and turnips. They are best eaten lightly steamed.

Other foods that help are these:

Curcuminoids (turmeric, curry)

Garlic and onions

Green tea (one to two cups a day)

High quality, sulfur-containing protein in eggs

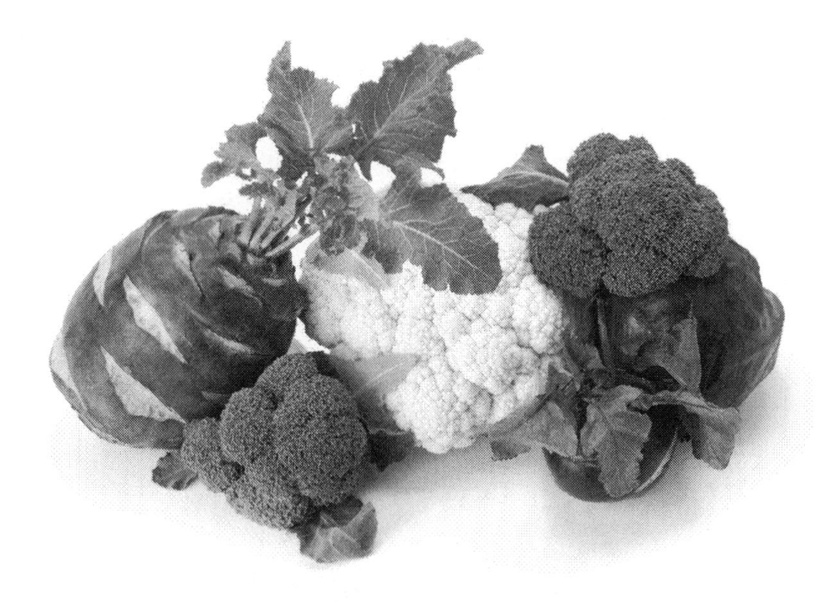

If you decide to do a four-day, ten-day, or twenty-one-day cleanse, which involves mostly liquids and a stricter diet, your doctor will give a good recommendation with a more specific menu plan.

Working with Your Doctor to Enhance Detoxification

In medically supervised detoxification programs, additional herbal supplements and phytonutrients may be used. They include alpha lipoic acid, bioactive whey protein, chelating agents, glutathione, and amino acids. Detoxifying from heavy metals is an important step on the road to health for many, and it needs to be done with an experienced and qualified health care practitioner. Proper testing preparation and care are needed in order for safe and effective heavy metal detoxification.

Below, you will find the steps I often recommend in order to prepare my patients for heavy metal detoxification. Specialized tests that assess your body's detoxification system may be ordered. These may include genetic testing for detoxification enzymes and heavy metals (including in the blood, urine, and hair). I want to reinforce that this must be done with a qualified health care practitioner. Once you have improved your health and optimized your detoxification system, you can begin to work to remove metals from your body through various approaches, including safe amalgam removal,[80] and the use of chelating agents, such as dimercaptosuccinic acid (DMSA). This medication will be prescribed; it is designed and approved for lead removal in children, but it is also effective against mercury and many other toxic metals.

Preparing for Detoxification

Below are the general guidelines I use with my patients. They should be done in collaboration with your doctor.

First, optimize your gut function by eliminating common food allergens. You may also take probiotics and enzymes for one to two months before detoxifying.

Optimize your nutritional status for detoxification by using healthy fats (omega 3 fats, olive oil, coconut oil) and minerals (particularly zinc and selenium, which help your body detoxify metals).

Enhance your liver's detoxification pathways, especially the sulfation and methylation pathways, by taking folate, B12, and B6, and by eating foods that contain sulfur, such as broccoli, collards, kale, daikon, radish, garlic, onion, and omega-3 eggs. Take supplements such as alpha lipoic acid and n-acetylcysteine.

Use herbal support for heavy metal detoxification, including alginate, cilantro, garlic, and milk thistle. Biofilam is a brand of seaweed from a pristine lake in New Zealand that has the highest level of alginate. You take it as capsules to clear your system of nuclear waste and heavy metals. You can learn more about this in the supplements section.

Start sauna therapy and make sure you take adequate electrolyte and mineral replacement to prevent dehydration and mineral loss from sweating.

Optimize metal elimination routes via your urine, stool, and sweat by drinking plenty of clean pure water, eating a diet high in plant fibers, and taking daily saunas for thirty minutes.

Sauna or Hyperthermia Therapy

Heat Therapies in Ancient Cultures

Sauna and heat therapies were used in ancient cultures for physical and spiritual purification. Most of us are familiar with the Native American sweat lodge, for example, as a tool for physical and spiritual purification. Scientific research is now validating practices such as the sweat lodge, used for thousands of years by Indigenous people for maintaining health. Sauna increases the rate of removing pollutants from fat. Sauna also increases the neuro-production of brain-derived growth factor and increases glutathione as well as B-endorphins. The storage site in the body for toxins is fat.

Dr. William L. Marcus, Chief Toxicologist for the US Environmental Protection Agency, stated, "It's a chronic exposure. That's why chemicals like dioxin, even in small amounts, are extremely dangerous. Unfortunately, the human body has no previous experience with these chemical and there is no natural machinery in the body to break them down, much less eliminate them."

If you recall what you learned in high school chemistry, some chemicals can readily dissolve in water and others dissolve only in oil bases. Every cell in our body has a fatty lipid cell membrane, and our brain in particular has a high fat content.[81]

Environmental Protection Agency Data

The Environmental Protection Agency has data demonstrating that sauna therapy increases excretion of heavy metals such as lead, mercury, and cadmium, and fat-soluble chemicals such as polychlorinated biphenyls (PCBs), heptachlor epoxide, and benzene, all three of which are found to cause cancer.[82]

For example, there was a study on one session of hyperthermia on twenty people, in which ten people were in a sauna, seven people in a steam room, and three people sweating through exercising. What came out of the sweat was the following: endosulfan (an insecticide), methoxychlor (an insecticide), DDT (an insecticide), DDE (the breakdown of DDT), Endrin (an insecticide, rodenticide, and pesticide), and perfluorinated compounds (an organic pollutant), all harmful compounds.[83]

In a Finnish study on 1,621 men, followed up in 24.7 years, having a sauna twice or three times a week reduced hypertension by 14 percent, and done four to seven times a week reduced it by 24 percent.[84]

In another study in Finland, 2,315 men whose ages ranged from 42 to 60 were followed for 20 years to look at their risk of developing dementia or Alzheimer's. The results showed that taking a sauna once a week lowered their risk by 22 percent and taking a sauna four to seven times a week lowered their risk of dementia by 75 percent.[85]

Follow These Guidelines for Safe Detoxification with a Sauna

The process of liberating fat-stored toxins through sweating must be done carefully and sometimes under a doctor's supervision to prevent complications.

If you are chronically ill or are taking medication, get your doctor's permission. Some individuals cannot tolerate the heat from a sauna or in a steam room. Waiting at least two months after a heart attack is best before having a sauna, according to a study of a hundred men.

- Find a health club or gym that has a sauna or a steam room.
- Consider building a sauna in your home; however, do your research beforehand to avoid using woods that off-gas toxins.
- For one-sixth the cost of a real wooden or glass sauna, you can get a portable sauna. My favorite brand is listed in the resources section.
- Drink at least 16 oz. of purified water *before* entering the sauna.
- Drink at least 16 oz. of purified water *after* the therapy.
- Start taking your sauna at 100°F, in short 10- to 20-minute increments.
- Sauna temperatures should be no higher than 140–150°F for those with environmental illness or a history of increased toxic exposures.
- If your blood pressure or respiratory rate increases ten points, get out.
- Stop if you experience a headache, nausea, heart rate increase of ten points, weakness, irregular heart rate, shortness of breath, dizziness, muscle cramps, spasms, or disorientation.

Maximize the Results of Your Sauna

To maximize the results of your sauna, follow these instructions:

- Take cold dips or rinses in a shower every 10 minutes. This drives the blood circulation from the periphery, where you were sweating, to the core, into the brain and kidneys. This will also help boost your mitochondria, which we will talk about in the next section.

- Prior to taking a sauna, exercise for 10–30 minutes to improve mobilization of chemicals or do a loofa sponge.
- Take Niacin (50–100 mg) prior to the sauna and titrate up by 50 mg each day. Stop titrating up when burning, flushing, or redness occurs. Benadryl will stop a reaction if it is unbearable.
- Take the enzyme Wobenzyme or Boluoke (can be purchased at a health food store) to clear stagnant sludge from the lymphatics.
- Replace the magnesium (200 mg twice or three times a day), zinc (15–25 mg), and calcium (800–1,200 mg) that is lost in the sweat.
- Take a daily detox cocktail of 1 to 2 packets of LivOn Labs vitamin C, 1 packet of LivOn Labs glutathione, and 300–600 mg of lipoic acid.
- Far infrared saunas run at a lower temperature, penetrate more deeply into the skin with more powerful detoxing, and may be more effective and more easily tolerated.
- Shower thoroughly with biodegradable soap, such as Dr. Bronner's, to clear the toxins off your skin from sweating after the sauna.

For intensive detoxification, daily saunas for six weeks can be helpful, with once-a-week maintenance therapy afterwards. There are some additional tips, as well as recommended saunas, in the resources section.

8 BOOSTING YOUR MITOCHONDRIA

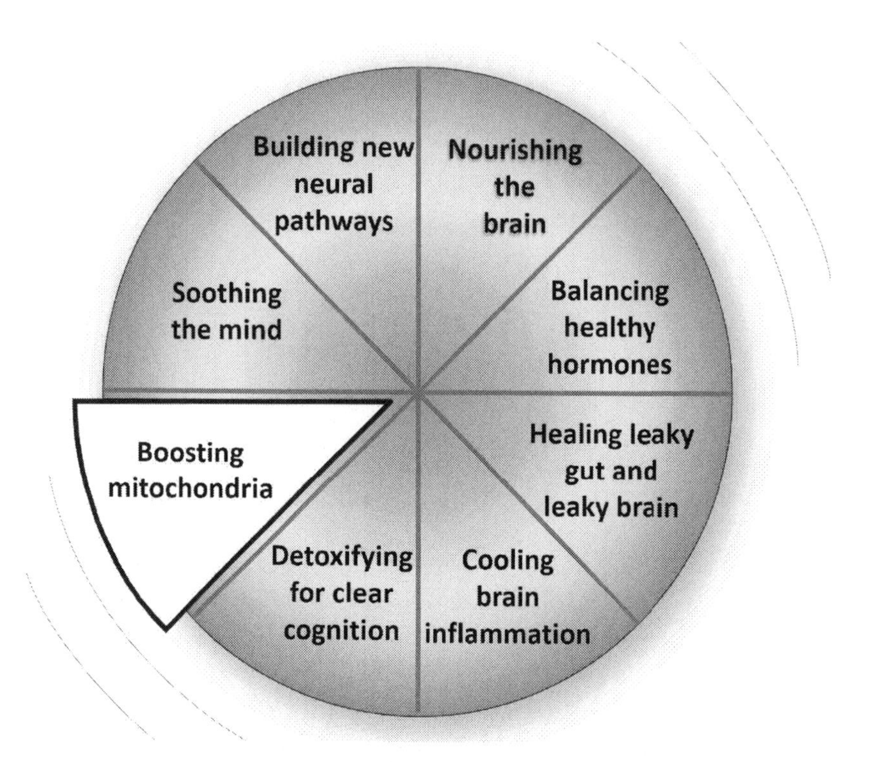

Where do we get the energy to actually run our body? Our energy comes from the tiny organelles called *mitochondria* that are inside every cell of our body. They are the energy generators for our bodies, forming cellular energy that comes in packets called *adenosine triphosphate* (ATP). ATP runs every energy function in the body, from enzyme reactions necessary for contracting the large muscle fibers (that allow us to sprint) to the minor muscles (that allow us to blink an eye). ATP also manufactures microscopic amounts of antioxidants. The process begins in the cell, with *glycolysis*, a process in which glucose is converted to acetyl coenzyme A through the Krebs cycle. Through an enzyme reaction called *oxidative phosphorylation*, electron donors transfer electrons to electron acceptors by using the electron transport chain. Energy is released when an electron is transferred to an acceptor such as oxygen. The mitochondria use the energy produced in the electron transport chain to manufacture ATP from adenosine diphosphate (ADP).

These are among the things that ATP does for us:

Boosts cellular repair for DNA

Helps synthesize brain chemicals and hormones

Helps the detox system in the liver, which breaks down certain pharmaceutical drugs and environmental toxins we breathe in, imbibe, or eat

Maintains optimal glutathione levels

MITOCHONDRIA

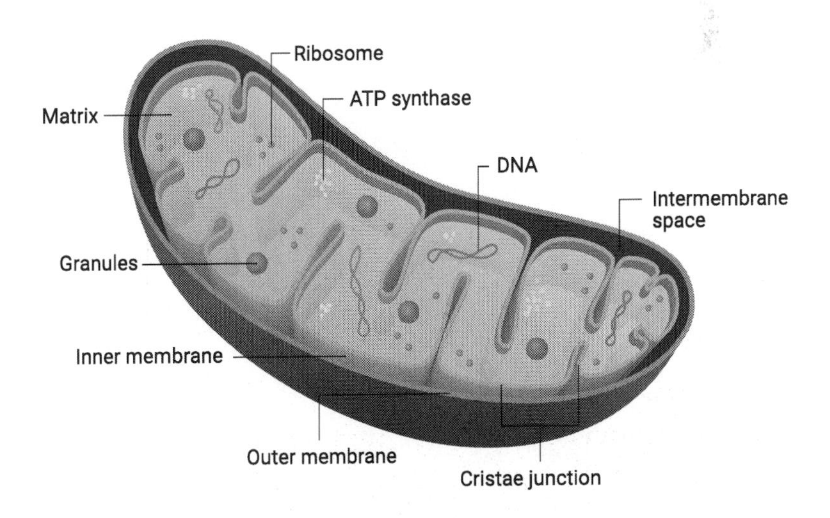

Generates peroxides for the immune system to release in oxidative bursts, thereby killing viruses and bacteria

Mitochondria take the carbohydrates, fats, and proteins that we eat and break them down into ATP. Specifically, they need glucose, fatty acids, and amino acids to do this. We have 500 to 2,000 mitochondria in each cell of our body. When our mitochondria are small in number, or when they shrink, we feel weak. When our mitochondria are larger in number and stronger, we feel strong. Through the process of *hormesis*, we can increase the number of mitochondria in our body and their size, thereby increasing our energy! Hormesis is a process whereby we put our body under stress. We can increase the size and number of our mitochondria through types of stress on the body, such as occasional fasting, or caloric restriction, as well as through intense bursts of physical exercise and muscle toning, or extremes in temperatures.

All the cells in our body have mitochondria. We could not live without them. Our skeletal muscles, however, actually contain the highest number of mitochondria per cell in our bodies. Therefore, the more we tone our muscles, the more mitochondria we grow. The mitochondria utilize 90 percent of our body's oxygen to make ATP.

These tiny organelles, the mitochondria, are often overlooked in the treatment of disease.

"Mitochondrial dysfunction's role in disease is particularly concerning given that the mitochondria of modern humans are subject to some assaults never experienced by people who lived before the early 1900s," write Chris D. Meletis, ND, and Kimberly Wilkes in the article "Mitochondria: Overlooking These Small Organelles Can Have Huge Clinical Consequences in Treating Virtually Every Disease."[86]

As you can see, our mitochondria are crucial to our operating and having energy to do the things we need to do in life.

Even though the mitochondria are often referred to as our powerhouses, like Superman, they also have a weakness. The DNA of mitochondria is more vulnerable to oxidative stress than DNA in other parts of our bodies, making it more vulnerable to malfunctioning—so much so that some physicians are calling this modern age we are living in "the Age of Mitochondrial Dysfunction." When our mitochondria lose their function or die, we see disease and problems with our memory, attention, and behavior. In the previous chapters I covered all of the things that create stress on our physiology, from physical trauma to the brain (as in a concussion) to plastics, heavy metals, food allergens, Roundup in our foods, and emotional stress. Oxidative stress and overexcitation to your brain can lead to elevated cortisol, which actually can lead to cell death, the *inability to retain information*, and more serious conditions such as ADHD and Alzheimer's. Toxins and stress overexcite your brain and send your nerve cells into chaos.

The wondrous thing about the human body is that it has built into it the natural desire to be in balance, which is called *homeostasis*. Since we come from nature, we act as nature does. We follow cyclical rhythms like day and night, activity and sleep. In balance, we experience health. All the systems in our body are in a constant process of doing checks and balances, a process called *allostasis*, meaning literally "maintaining stability through change." If we go outside that range or if our load of stressors becomes too great, we compromise our health. There are short-term stress effects, such as from burning your finger on a stove or candle, which may take a few days to heal, or getting delayed because of a traffic jam; and there are long-term effects, such as from hip arthritis over many years, which leads to requiring a hip replacement to relieve pain and increase mobility. When we lose our balance, illness finds a way in. Fortunately, the body has the means to protect itself against overexcitation. Good nutrition plays a key role here. For example, magnesium protects the N-methyl-D-aspartate (NMDA) receptor from being overexcited by glutamate—the neurotransmitter that normally flips the receptor switch on. Zinc and green tea act as brakes on the overstimulation of the NMDA receptor.

Aging and the Mitochondria

Aging is one of the key drivers of mitochondrial dysfunction. We lose half of our mitochondria from age twenty to forty and a quarter from age forty to seventy. This happens in people who don't carry out certain practices. Ari Whitten, founder of the Energy Blueprint and an exercise physiologist, sports medicine expert, nutritionist, and performance enhancement specialist, promotes the body-stressing process called hormesis as a profoundly positive tool to help slow the detrimental effects of aging on the mitochondria. Hormesis is essentially stressing the body temporarily in intermittent burst of extreme temperature changes, hypoxic exposure, demand on muscles when fasting, and intermittent fasting. The genes of the mitochondria are referred to as *sirtuins*. These genes control genetic, biochemical, and cellular pathways involved in aging. Multiplying the expression of these genes through hormesis is thought to increase longevity. With age, mitochondrial oxidative phosphorylation becomes less efficient.[87] One way to amplify the expression of the genes of mitochondria and actually make *more* mitochondria in your body is through this process of hormesis.

Neuro-nutrients: Boosting Your Mitochondria and Your Brain Power

Fortunately, the branches of medicine called *integrative medicine* and *functional medicine* have been studying the relationship between the human genome, nutrition, and health for decades. The term coined from this aspect of medicine is *nutrigenomics*. What is being discovered is that high doses of natural nutrients normally found in our food can protect our mitochondria from oxidative stress. This class of nutrients is called antioxidants. Antioxidants are an important part of helping us achieve and keep a sharp, clear mind and optimal energy.

Supplements to Boost Mitochondria

Some supplements to boost mitochondria include the following:

Alpha-lipoic acid

Coenzyme Q10

L-carnitine

N-acetylcysteine (NAC)

Nicotinamide riboside

One randomized, double-blind clinical trial that used a combination of creatine monohydrate, coenzyme Q10, and alpha-lipoic acid lowered markers of oxidative stress in mitochondrial diseases.[88]

Also important to mitochondrial health is L-carnitine, because it heals the transfer of long-chain fatty acids available for energy production that might otherwise result in symptoms such as myalgia and muscle weakness.[89]

Modern medicine has created a mindset of "one pill per condition." Nutrients naturally come in food, which has a mixture of vitamins, minerals, and macronutrients working together synergistically. The solution cannot be to take one nutrient, because nutrients work together in teams. No matter how good that one vitamin or mineral is, it needs to be part of a team of players for it to function properly. It's important to change that "one pill per condition" mindset when working with nutrigenomics.

Superfoods to Improve Mitochondria

Based on findings of the Institute of Functional Medicine, here is a list of superfoods most supportive to improving the health and function of your mitochondria:

Almonds
Arugula
Avocado
Beef
Blackberries
Blueberries
Bok choy
Broccoli and broccoli sprouts
Brussels sprouts
Buffalo
Cabbage
Cauliflower
Extra virgin olive oil
Kale
Kohlrabi
Mustard and turnip greens
Pomegranate
Raspberries
Spinach
Strawberries
Turmeric
Virgin coconut oil
Watercress
Wild Pacific salmon

The Benefits of Exercising

Exercise is one of the single most powerful habits for your health. Exercising enhances energy and memory and boosts mitochondria.

Exercise does many things: helps balance and even out stress hormone levels, reduces oxidative stress, reduces the effects of emotional stress, increases blood circulation and oxygenation to all parts of the body, and increases lean muscle mass. There are different types of exercise. Cardiovascular exercise increases the circulation of oxygenated blood to all parts of the body. Lifting weights and doing muscle toning exercises that involve a certain number of repetitions will not only bulk up your muscles but also your mitochondria! People who increase lean muscle mass through toning the muscles will simultaneously increase the number of mitochondria, their volume and their size! This results in more ATP and essentially, you feeling more energetic! Exercise also helps you sleep at night, thereby recuperating your brain. Exercise helps keep insulin levels down and blood sugar levels even. Exercise boosts the immune system. Finally, exercise has been shown to help produce brain-derived nerve factor (BDNF), helping the brain with memory.

During the office visit with your doctor that is part of the Regenerate Your Brain Program, you will come up with an exercise plan. The rule of thumb is thirty minutes of movement a day; at the very least, ten minutes twice a day if you cannot find thirty minutes of time in a block. Ideally, it is good to have different levels of intensity of exercise.

A recent revolutionary understanding of exercise for the brain has shown that even a seven-minute workout raises BDNF, the chemical that helps the brain with memory. Not surprisingly, it is called the *seven-minute workout*. It was reviewed in a *New York Times* article on May 9, 2013.

Here are sections of that article:

> *An article in the May–June 2013 issue of the American College of Sports Medicine's* Health & Fitness Journal *reports that "In 12 exercises deploying only body weight, a chair and a wall,* [the seven-minute workout] *fulfills the latest mandates for high-intensity effort, which essentially combines a long run and a visit to the weight room into about seven minutes of steady discomfort—all of it based on science.*

"There's very good evidence" that high-intensity interval training provides "many of the fitness benefits of prolonged endurance training but in much less time," says Chris Jordan, the director of exercise physiology at the Human Performance Institute in Orlando, Fla., and co-author of the article.[90]

Scientists at McMaster University in Hamilton, Ontario (among other reputable institutions), have shown that even a few minutes of training at an intensity approaching your maximum capacity produces molecular changes within muscles comparable to those of several hours of running or bike riding.

Interval training, though, requires intervals; the extremely intense activity must be intermingled with brief periods of recovery. In the program outlined by Chris Jordan and his colleagues, this recovery is provided in part by a ten-second rest between exercises. But even more, he says, it's accomplished by alternating an exercise that emphasizes the large muscles in the upper body with those in the lower body. During the intermezzo, the unexercised muscles have a moment to, metaphorically, catch their breath, which makes the order of the exercises important. The exercises should be performed in rapid succession, allowing thirty seconds for each while, throughout, the intensity hovers at about an 8 on a discomfort scale of 1 to 10, Mr. Jordan says. Those seven minutes should be, in a word, unpleasant. The upside is, after seven minutes, you're done.[91] Here is a video of the seven-minute exercise.[92]

Exercising your physical body is not the only kind of exercise that can be helpful to the brain. You also want to engage your intellectual functions to encourage the maintenance of neural circuitry.

Researchers at the Mayo Clinic reported in the January 2010 issue of *JAMA Neurology* that older people who engage in mentally stimulating activities like games, crafts, and computer use have a lower risk of developing mild cognitive impairment, often a precursor to dementia. Also helpful is if players participate with other people; social engagement has repeatedly been shown to benefit health and longevity.[93]

The researchers, led by Dr. Yonas E. Geda, a psychiatrist and behavioral neurologist at Mayo, followed nearly 2,000 cognitively normal people 70 or older for an average of four years. After adjusting the results for sex, age, and education level, they found that computer use decreased the participants' risk of cognitive impairment by 30 percent, engaging in crafts decreased it by 28 percent, and playing games decreased it by 22 percent.

Dr. Geda said that those who performed such activities at least once or twice a week experienced less cognitive decline than those who did the same activities at most only three times a month.

Hyperbaric Oxygen Therapy

Many people have never heard of hyperbaric oxygen therapy (HBOT) before, so let me explain a little more about what it is, how it works, and how I got introduced to it personally. In medical school, we were taught very little about HBOT. In fact, we learned about it only as a form of emergency medicine for divers to treat "the bends." Also known as decompression sickness, the bends are caused by rapid changes in pressure during scuba diving. It occurs when a diver surfaces too fast and dissolved gases (mainly nitrogen) come out of solution in the bloodstream, forming gas bubbles in the body.

I'd like to come back to my own personal story about my brain injury here. If you recall, in my forties, I had three infections in my brain, which I received from a tick bite while hiking in Muir Woods, California. For four months I was treated for these infections with triple antibiotics and herbal medicines. After six weeks on those antibiotics I felt radically better; my fevers, sore throat, and tremors all disappeared, never to return. However, my cognitive speed and endurance were greatly diminished. This diminishment showed up in my life as the inability to multitask, which made being a doctor very hard. Multitasking included driving somewhere new and looking at my GPS, or taking typed notes while someone was talking, or fetching an object I needed while thinking of my to-do list. Balls got dropped.

I had set up a life in which operating cognitively at half throttle simply was not an option. I was very fortunate at the time to know about HBOT, as I worked at an HBOT facility as the prescribing physician. I never thought, however, that I would benefit from going in the chamber myself. But I knew of many patients who had come to us with cognitive decline after a long-standing illness and got radically better after a series of HBOT sessions.

It didn't take much convincing for me to try a full course of HBOT on myself. What happened was astounding. A full course of therapy is forty sessions, each one lasting ninety minutes. In the thirty-fifth session, I was simply relaxing in the chamber when the oxygen went to the part of my brain that had been scarred when I fell off my bike at fourteen. I knew this because at the time I had also cut my left eyebrow wide open and gouged my left knee, both of which needed stiches. While I was in the chamber on that thirty-fifth session, I felt those areas as if they were swelling up. An area of my brain was being oxygenated and re-creating a body memory that was over 20 years old. My eyes teared up from the scare of the fall. This happened completely spontaneously. After the completion of my forty sessions, I felt as though my brain was operating twenty times faster. I felt the sharpness and speed of my intellectual abilities that I had in my college years return.

Stories like mine and plenty of others are why at our medical clinic we refer to HBOT as "Superman without the cape." High concentrations of oxygen can produce miracles when properly administered. Hyperbaric oxygen is 100 percent medical-grade oxygen administered under pressure. It is a medical treatment that requires a doctor's prescription. Even though our brain only weighs two pounds, it uses 20 percent of our body's oxygen! In fact, we know that high levels of oxygen under pressure affect the expression of over eight thousand genes! One of the most powerful ways to rejuvenate the brain is with HBOT, because it provides between fourteen and twenty times more oxygen to your brain cells while you are in the chamber than you receive through normal breathing.[94]

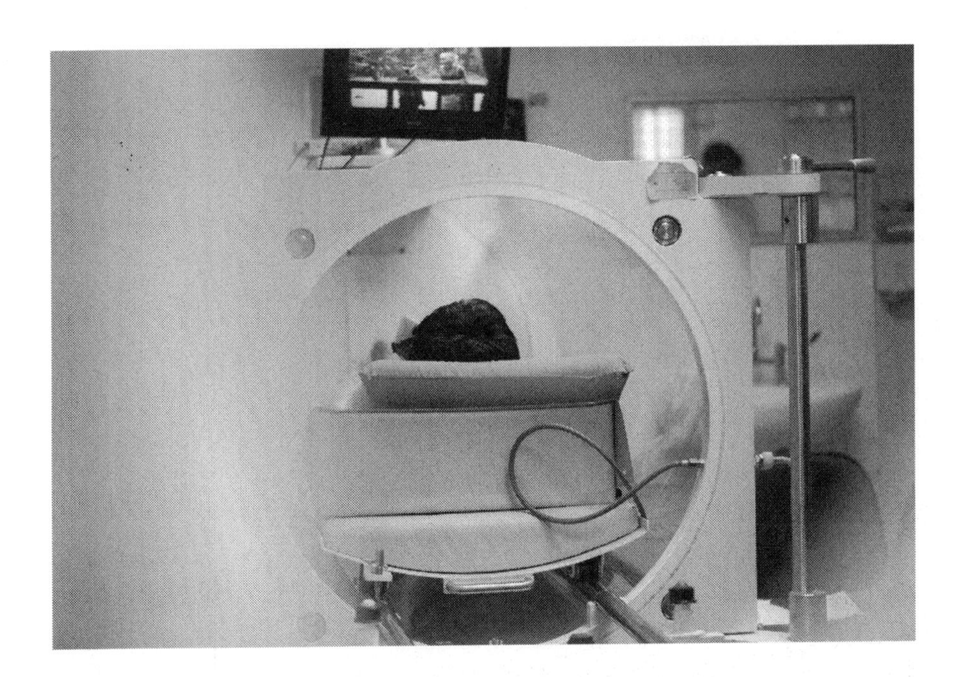

HBOT Awakens Oxygen-Starved Tissue

Since our air is only 20 percent oxygen and HBOT delivers 100 percent oxygen in a chamber under pressure, a higher-than-normal amount of oxygen diffuses into the tissue. A gas—in this case, oxygen—under pressure increases its absorption into a physical medium, be it air, blood, or liquid. In the HBOT chamber, the pressure ranges from 1.3 to 2.8 atmospheres absolute, providing a much-increased tissue level of oxygen. What we are breathing right now is considered 1 atmosphere absolute, which is technically 760 mmHg of pressure. This is just like nitrogen bubbles pressurized into water, which create soda. This physics law is called Dalton's law of partial pressure. What you are breathing right now as you read this is 20 percent oxygen at one atmospheric pressure, or sea level. One atmosphere of pressure is abbreviated as 1 ATA. We don't really feel the "pressure," because we were born, have grown up, slept, eaten, and walked around in it our entire lives.

Oxygen is normally delivered to tissues by the red blood cells. Right now, for example, you're breathing oxygen in and it is being absorbed by your red blood cells in the alveoli, the small air sacs in the lungs. There are thousands of alveoli in the lungs, capturing oxygen from our breath and transporting it into our blood. Once our blood is oxygenated, it is a healthy, vital bright red, and when it has run out of oxygen it turns blue. One of the unique aspects of hyperbaric oxygen is that it creates such a high amount of oxygen in the blood that some of it detaches from the red blood cells and travels into the plasma and through the capillary walls into the tissue beyond the capillaries. This means that oxygen is reaching areas where there are no capillaries! This is a completely unique feature of HBOT. In fact, so much oxygen can course through the capillary wall and into low-oxygen-level tissue that after weeks of therapy a whole new blood vessel can be formed where there was not one previously.

Gretl Lam, BA, et al. write in their article "Hyperbaric Oxygen Therapy: Exploring the Clinical Evidence," published in the April 2017 edition of *Advances in Skin and Wound Care Journal:*

> *Improved neovascularization occurs through both local and distant processes. Locally, reactive oxygen species and reactive nitrogen species signal an increased production of wound growth factors, such as vascular endothelial growth factor (the most specific factor for neovascularization), transforming growth factor β1, and angiopoietin 2. Endothelial cells exposed to hyperbaric oxygen exhibit enhanced capillary tube formation and enhanced oxidative stress resistance.*
>
> *Although hypoxia stimulates neovascularization, chronic hypoxia actually inhibits new vessel formation. For this reason, hyperoxia induced by HBOT promotes neovascularization and healing of chronic wounds. In addition, it is important to distinguish between oxidative stress and oxygen toxicity. Excessive reactive oxygen species are associated with harmful effects; however, studies have shown that the body's antioxidant*

> *defenses protect against the limited number of reactive oxygen species generated by HBOT treatment sessions.*

HBOT Is a Remedy for the Toxic Effects of Impaired Circulation

Neurosurgeon Russell Blaylock, MD, wrote this in *The Blaylock Wellness Report* (vol. 15, no. 11, November 2018, page 4):

> *To understand the value of HBOT, you need to understand a little about medical biology. Most people know that oxygen is carried to tissues and organs by major blood vessels. But the actual introduction of oxygen into the tissues—along with removal of carbon dioxide—takes place in what are referred to as micro vessels: arterioles and, primarily, capillaries.*

Many of our diseases can result in impaired microcirculation. This is the physiological underpinning of diabetes, in which the circulation is impaired by microvessel damage and all organs are affected: there is poor wound healing, visual blindness, and kidney failure, as well as loss of sensation or nerve pain in the nerves in the extremities.

Dr. Blaylock continues:

> *In addition, hypoxia-induced inflammation activates special immune cells in the brain called microglia. When that happens, there is a buildup of two brain-destructive compounds—inflammatory cytokines and excitotoxins. The interaction of these two compounds leads to an extremely destructive process called immune excitotoxicity. As we age, our bodies become progressively more inflamed. This means they are becoming progressively more hypoxic. This is where HBOT can be beneficial. It has been shown that HBOT treatments increase microcirculation not just during treatments, but permanently.*

HBOT Resuscitates the Mitochondria

Oxygen is profoundly helpful to our mitochondria, the powerhouses of our cells. Oxygen enters the mitochondria and goes through an electron transport chain to make ATP, which fuels every cellular and enzymatic reaction in the body. The DNA of the mitochondria in the brain are more susceptible to damage than in other parts of our body. Improving mitochondria function leads to more energy, which then translates to less brain fog.

The following is from "Oxygen Administration Selectively Enhances Cognitive Performance in Healthy Young Adults," published in 1998 by Moss et al. in *Psychopharmacology* 138(1):27-33[95]:

> *Oxygen administration significantly improved performance on several measures of attention and vigilance. Simple reaction time, choice reaction time, digit vigilance reaction time and picture recognition reaction time were improved in a manner which depended on the duration of oxygen inspired.*[96]

In addition, a study looking at chronic, traumatic brain injuries with and without post-traumatic stress disorder (PTSD) showed that in sixteen male patients who had received thirty HBOT sessions at 1.5 ATA for sixty minutes, each had an average 50 percent reduction in depression, 40 percent reduction in anxiety, and an increase in IQ of 14 percent.

There is also a milestone study of a case of reversal of Alzheimer's in a woman at the early age of fifty-eight. She had been experiencing cognitive decline for five years prior, with a rapid progression of dementia in the eight months prior to receiving HBOT. An eight-week course of HBOT reversed her symptomatic decline! After the HBOT she reported improved memory and concentration, decreased disorientation, and less frustration; in addition, her anxiety was gone. Her cognitive clarity sustained itself for at least twenty-two months. The brain scans showed 6.5 to 38.0 percent improvement in overall brain metabolism. This is the first brain imaging study to document improvements in brain metabolism in a patient with Alzheimer's disease.[97]

HBOT is a revolutionary treatment for the underlying pathophysiology of traumatic brain injury, concussion, stroke, dementia, and many other neurological and systemic diseases. When a person has a stroke or an ischemic neurological event, there is a penumbra around the area of brain damage, an area that is stunned and idling but not actually dead. Oxygen will awaken these brain cells, salvaging them. They may be idling for many years. Oxygen revives the mitochondria in these cells and increases stem cell production.

A team of researchers set out to answer the question "What are the most reliable predictors of Alzheimer's disease?" Wouldn't you want to know that? In an enormous undertaking, they looked at over 7,700 brain images, measurements of plasma, and cerebrospinal fluid biomarkers and did a multifactorial analysis, which they published in June 2016. Taking into consideration all possible causes of dementia (such as metabolic, vascular, functional activity at rest, structural properties, cognitive integrity, and amyloid-B deposition), what they discovered is that low blood flow is the number one brain imaging predictor that a person will develop Alzheimer's disease.[98]

Low blood flow means not getting enough oxygen to the tissues. When the brain doesn't get enough oxygen, the cells in the brain begin to fail. In fact, we can live a week without food and several days without water but only four minutes without oxygen!

HBOT can help numerous conditions. Regarding the brain, HBOT can help with these situations and conditions:

Alzheimer's disease
Autism[99]
Carbon monoxide poisoning
Cerebral palsy[100]
Lyme disease
Migraine
Multiple sclerosis[101]

Sports injuries
Stroke
Traumatic brain injury[102]
Vascular dementia[103]

HBOT and the Stimulation of New Tissue Growth through Stem Cells

When oxygen at a level up to twenty times more than usual courses through the body, it stimulates the release of stem cells from bone marrow. Stem cells are undifferentiated pluripotent cells that are capable of becoming any cell. They come from either our fat tissue or bone marrow. These cells have the potential to become heart, brain, liver, or bone cells, as they are capable of differentiating into specific cell types. In fact, one HBOT session at twice the atmospheric pressure (2.0 ATA) for sixty minutes will double the number of stem cells; twenty sessions will increase the stem cells sixteen-fold. These stem cells can go on to become brain, heart, liver, or joint tissue.

HBOT, DNA Signaling, and the Ocean Safari

The oxygen component of HBOT acts as a DNA signaling agent, something that was discovered in 1997 and proven in multiple studies over the next eleven years. Very few things in life actually signal our bodies to develop and grow. When you really ponder oxygen, not only is it the third most abundant element in the universe, it was the initiator of life as we know it on earth. The planet formed 4.6 billion years ago and was devoid of oxygen. Our oceans were brown with iron ore. When we think of oxygen, we think of the sky as the main source, but oxygen was first created in the ocean, turning it from brown to blue by the action of cyanobacteria (blue-green algae) 3.5 billion years ago. Cyanobacteria were the first forms of life. Living in the ocean, they used sunshine, water, and carbon dioxide (CO_2) to produce oxygen through the process of photosynthesis. Oxygen thus came from the ocean and filled the air for about one billion years, until 2.45 billion years ago, when there was enough oxygen in the air for animal life to evolve from unicellular organisms that had been dominating the scene. It's no surprise then that oxygen under pressure (deep life in the ocean is under heavy water pressure) signals genes coded for growth and repair.

In his *Townsend Letter* article of April 2018, Paul Harch, MD, elucidates how HBOT actually stimulates tissue growth[104]:

> *The question remained, how do repetitive administrations of intermittent increases in pressure and oxygen reverse pathophysiology and stimulate tissue growth? Tissue growth requires replication of DNA. In 1997, Siddiqui et al. argued that the oxygen component of HBOT was a DNA signaling agent. Multiple publications confirmed this concept in the next 11 years, culminating in the demonstration that a single HBOT at the pressure used for diabetic foot wounds and radiation wounds up-or-down regulated the expression of 8,101 of the known 19-20,000 protein-coding genes in the human genome. The largest clusters of up-regulated genes were the anti-inflammatory genes and those that coded for growth and repair hormone. The largest clusters of down-regulated genes were the pro-inflammatory genes and apoptotic genes which are genes that regulate cell death. Further work showed the differential gene effects of pressure and oxygen, whereby different and similar clusters of neuronal genes are affected by different pressures and different amounts of hyperoxia. In essence, during hyperbaric therapy physicians are playing a symphony with patients' gene expression, the music of which is determined by the various pressures and amounts of hyperoxia to which the patient is exposed.*

HBOT is proven to reduce cerebral edema and neuro-inflammation, increase oxygen saturation to the brain, promote new blood vessel growth, generate new stem cells, and reactivate idling neurons.

What Is the Procedure of HBOT Like?

The procedure of receiving HBOT treatment is straightforward. There are two types of chambers. A multi-place chamber is the size of a large room and accommodates as many as twenty people. Each person puts on a mask that delivers 100 percent oxygen. A mono-place chamber, which looks like a healing cocoon, holds one person. Their entire body receives the 100 percent oxygen and they do not wear a mask.

The person enters the special hyperbaric chamber that provides oxygen under pressure. Inside the chamber, the oxygen pressure is higher than at sea level, generally at 1.4 times atmospheric pressure or higher. It is an extremely pleasant experience of lying down, relaxing, and breathing fresh, 100-percent pure oxygen.

You may relax or rest during your sessions. Some centers, such as ours, show movies, provide music for relaxation or meditation, or deliver educational material. As the treatment proceeds, your eardrums respond to changes in pressure and you will begin to experience a sensation of fullness in the ears, much as you might do on an airplane. At this time, you may sip water, yawn, or perform any other needed exercise to clear your ears.

At our facility you are never unattended. You can speak to the hyperbaric technician at any time through a two-way intercom. The hyperbaric oxygen treatments will last sixty to ninety minutes, depending on your physician's prescription, which varies in time spent and depth of pressure in the chamber, based on which condition you are being treated for. Your physician will prescribe your dosage of HBOT based on your history and current condition.

If you have vascular dementia or a traumatic brain injury, such as one or more concussions, consider taking a course of HBOT. Find an HBOT physician or facility near you, as this therapy requires daily treatments of one to two hours for at least five days a week for two weeks or more.

HBOT Testimonials

You may be interested to watch these three video testimonials[105] about HBOT from individuals whom I treated at the Advanced Hyperbaric Recovery of Marin: "Hyperbaric Oxygen Therapy for Post-Concussion," "Rapid Recovery from Concussion and Trauma," and "ICU Nurse suffering from post-stroke effects regains quality of life with Hyperbaric Oxygen Therapy!" Each of these patients suffered a brain injury.

Basic Diet Plan for Boosting Mitochondria

The Regenerate Your Brain Program includes a diet plan based on thirty years of research on optimal nutrition for our body's energy generators, our mitochondria. You will receive this diet plan during your office visit with your doctor. This diet plan will take care of most of your needs. This short list of foods (it is not comprehensive; you will get the comprehensive list as part of your first office visit) suggests the ones you want to focus on to boost your energy factories, as mentioned earlier in this chapter:

Almonds
Arugula
Avocado
Beef
Blackberries
Blueberries
Bok choy
Broccoli and broccoli sprouts
Brussels sprouts
Buffalo
Cabbage

Cauliflower
Extra virgin olive oil
Kale
Kohlrabi
Mustard and turnip greens
Pomegranate
Raspberries
Spinach
Strawberries
Turmeric
Virgin coconut oil
Watercress
Wild Pacific salmon

Eating vegetables and fruits that are varied in color is optimal. The richer and darker in color the fruit or vegetable, the more potent the antioxidants and energy boosters in the food. Remember, eat a rainbow diet of colors and you will have loads of energy.

Crucial for your mitochondria is the inclusion of exercise. The smartphone app for the seven-minute workout that raises your level of BDNF is called "Scientific 7-Minute Workout." Other important exercises for the brain include learning a new language, practicing math, taking a partner dance class, and playing speed-and-accuracy computer games such as such as Posit Science's *Brain HQ* or Lumosity's brain games.

Supplements for Boosting Energy

Certain *nutraceuticals* (fortified foods that benefit health) protect these precious batteries in our body and give them more energy. The special nutrients listed below enhance your ATP production when your mitochondria are under conditions of stress, toxicity, and aging. These nutrients can dramatically improve mitochondrial function and protect the mitochondria from damage. The most important of these are as follows:

Acetyl-L-carnitine, 500 mg twice a day. L-carnitine is an amino acid that produces energy by transporting fatty acids into the cell's mitochondria.

Alpha-lipoic acid (ALA), 600–1800 mg daily. ALA is also a nutrient cofactor involved in mitochondrial function, thus supporting energy production in the cells. At these higher amounts it can help maintain mental sharpness. In addition to being an important antioxidant in both fat-soluble and water-soluble tissues, ALA also helps recycle other antioxidants, including glutathione, another essential antioxidant for liver detoxification.

Coenzyme Q10 (CoQ10, also known as Ubiquinol), 100 mg a day. CoQ10 is an enzyme that lodges into the complexes on the electron transport chain in the mitochondria, speeding up the production of ATP.

Nicotinamide riboside (NAD) 250–500 mg twice a day. This boosts cellular repair for DNA; is involved in synthesis of brain chemicals and hormones; increases the rate of ATP production in the mitochondria; maintains glutathione levels, which helps detoxification; and generates peroxides for release in oxidative burst by the immune system, which kills viruses and bacteria. With aging, our NAD decreases by 50 percent every twenty years. As you age you need more NAD.

Supplement that creates new brain connections

Lion's mane is a mushroom that raises brain derived nerve growth factor (BDNF) in the brain. BDNF helps create healthy new brain connections and works like magic to reverse brain shrinkage.

Researchers at the University of California, San Diego, looked at the brains of monkeys who were in the human age-equivalent of their late sixties. More than half of their brain cells had shrunk by *at least* 10 percent. But the remaining brain cells had shrunk so much, they were barely visible at all—withered away like tiny deflated balloons. When the researchers injected BDN7 into the monkeys' brains, the withered cells "re-inflated" and sprang back to life. In fact, the researchers were able to detect more than 90 percent of what would be considered normal for a much younger monkey. Natural ways to increase BDNF are physical exercise and cognitive training.[106]

Lab Work

An organic acid test is often used to diagnose mitochondrial dysfunction. Organic acids are produced as a result of the breakdown of proteins, carbohydrates, and fats. The presence or elevation of specific organic acids can serve as a marker for mitochondrial abnormalities or can indicate exposure to toxins that may be harmful to the mitochondria. Organic acid tests can measure a marker for CoQ10 deficiency, impairment of oxidative phosphorylation, and a functional deficiency in carnitine.[107]

Your physician can help you with lab work to reveal your antioxidant levels, by testing your blood, hair, or urine. The lab work results can direct you to optimize your nutrition. Getting a metabolic tune-up is not only possible but necessary for most of us. Follow the Regenerate Your Brain Program and add in a few supplements to boost your mitochondria.

9 | SOOTHING YOUR MIND

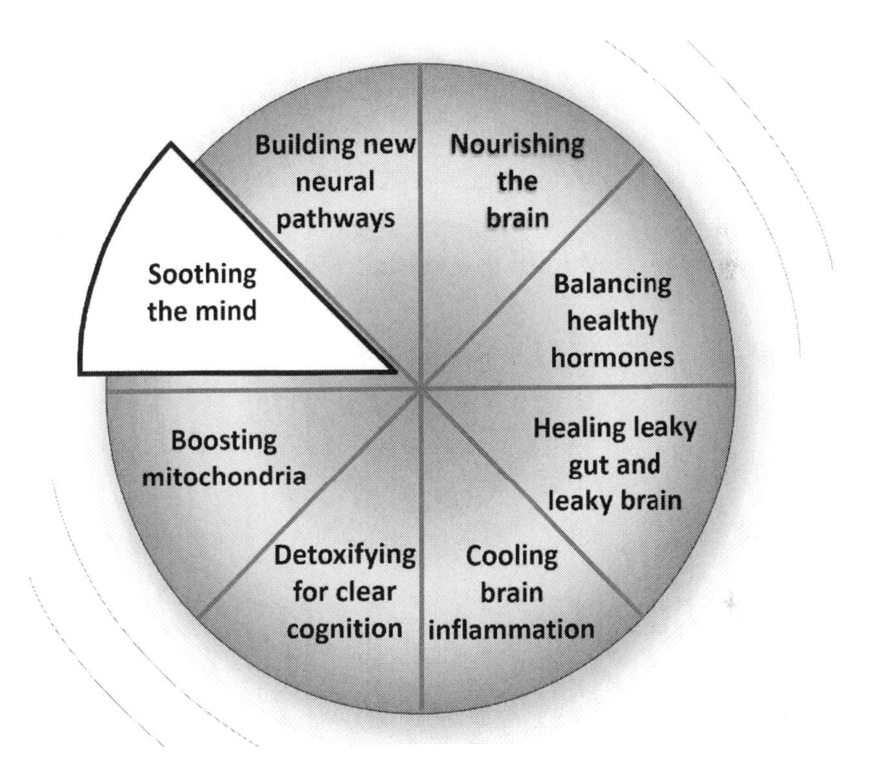

Sleep and Deep Rest

When I first taught students about the treatment of memory issues, I was told by the senior teaching physician, "If you have a patient who complains of memory loss, tell them to sleep eight hours a night for two weeks in a row and see if their memory loss continues." You should note that in most cases, memory loss is no longer there. In the book *Why We Sleep: Unlocking the Power of Sleep and Dreams*, author Matthew Walker, PhD, explains that during sleep, our brain actually moves short-term memories into long-term memory storage, creating more space for new memories and learning to take place. If restorative sleep is lacking, our stress hormone levels go up, while our hippocampus atrophies and shrinks. Lack of sleep causes poor memory retrieval, overwhelm, and self-doubt as hippocampal function degrades. It doesn't take much convincing of the scientific facts for us to accept that sleep loss impairs our memory, as most of us have experienced this first-hand. Sleep disturbances are also strongly associated with the impaired release of growth or trophic factors such as brain-derived neurotrophic factor and insulin-like growth factor-1. Optimal function of growth factors protects mood, staves off depression, and maintains neuroplasticity. Keep in mind that the most important population for requiring healthy sleep are our children, as their brains are still developing and growing. School-aged children require between nine and twelve hours of sleep a night, according to health reports.

A List of Issues That Affect Sleep

Many issues affect our sleep. Here are some:

- Excessive caffeine, which suppresses melatonin production by the cells of the pineal gland.
- Too much alcohol, because it blocks deep REM sleep (sleep with rapid eye movements), which is the most restorative type of sleep. This issue is more pronounced in women, who have smaller livers that are unable to process alcohol as efficiently.
- Not enough exercise. Adding just fifteen to twenty minutes of exercise to your day gets your circulation going and allows your body to wind down more successfully during nighttime hours.
- Not getting outside. Being outside in nature, even if just for twenty minutes a day, can help.

- Hormone fluctuations in women who are going through menopause. Estrogen fluctuations can cause night sweats, whereas progesterone is a natural anxiolytic by binding to some of the GABA binding sites. A Belgian double-blind, placebo-controlled study found that women who took 300 mg of oral progesterone before bed got to sleep faster, slept better, and had higher levels of growth hormone and even more stable blood levels of thyroid hormone.[108]
- Unresolved emotions of sadness, fear, regret, perfectionism, and guilt can disrupt sleep.
- A lack of growth hormones. Human growth hormone is released in the first deep-sleep episode of the night. When adequate levels are released, this phase of sleep is associated with deep body-mind rejuvenation. Growth hormone is essential for restorative sleep and vice versa. Growth hormone naturally lowers as we age. Taking a sauna can naturally increase our growth hormone levels.

How to Sleep Better Naturally

The obvious solutions to some of the items on the list of issues would be to cut out some of the above-mentioned poor-sleep inducers, for instance, to cut back on caffeine and alcohol. Generally, I recommend no caffeine after noon. Skip the evening iced tea or coffee after dinner, and if you want a hot beverage, switch to mint, rooibos, or chamomile tea. Cutting out alcohol in the late evening also helps; or only have alcohol one or two nights a week.

If you are a menopausal woman, hormones, such as progesterone, can be a lifesaver. Taking melatonin is another great option. Melatonin is naturally secreted by the brain's pineal gland in response to cycles of light and darkness, regulating your ability to stay in sync with the time of day. Sleep in as dark a room as possible. You can get night blinds to put on your windows to keep any daylight from coming in, and be sure to turn off electrical devices in the room. Natural melatonin secretion is dysregulated by light at night, shift work, and seasonal affective disorder, which occurs during dark winter days. Melatonin is also a major antioxidant for the brain. The usual dose is 0.5–3.0 mg taken half an hour before bedtime. Melatonin can safely be used with other bioidentical hormones and even with hormone-blocking medications. Melatonin does not increase the risk of cancer; in fact, it's a powerful aid in reducing the chances of brain cancer.

Supplements

Supplements that can help with sleep are these:

> **Liposomal GABA**—this goes through the blood-brain barrier and quiets the central nervous system, acting as a natural *anxiolytic* (a drug to relieve anxiety). Taking 500 mg of GABA thirty minutes before bed is helpful, especially for anxiety.
>
> **Magnesium**—300 mg helps with muscle tension and insomnia in general.
>
> **Magnolia bark**—this lowers cortisol at night, increasing the amount of time in deep REM sleep.
>
> **Melatonin**—0.5–3.0 mg thirty minutes before bedtime mimics the natural melatonin your pineal gland produces when it becomes dark outside. This is an excellent choice for recovering from jet lag and if you are unable to be in a dark room to sleep.
>
> **Valerian**—this bitter-tasting liquid is helpful initially for falling asleep. Take 150–300 mg standardized to 0.8 percent valerenic acid one hour before pulling up the covers.

Avoid Sleeping Pills

This may seem counterintuitive, but I recommend you avoid sleeping pills. Why wouldn't you take sleeping pills to sleep? I can't tell you how many patients I have had whose energy level and brain health has been poorly affected by taking sleeping pills for years.

Devaki Lindsey Berkson, MA, DC, wrote an article for the February–March 2019 *Townsend Letter* entitled "New Whys and Ways to Sleep Better, Especially After 40." Citing articles in *Sleep*, *BMJ Open*, and the *Journal of Clinical Sleep Medicine*, she claimed that even taking less than eighteen sleep hypnotics in a single year has been linked to dying prematurely from all-cause mortality.

The sleeping pill fix is not worth it. If you take them, use them for the shortest time possible while you fix the root issues causing your insomnia. Sometimes doctors say that antihistamine drugs for allergies cause less drowsiness and are less dangerous than sleeping pills, so why not take them? Not true. Antihistamine medicines block *acetylcholine*, which lowers neurotransmitters and is crucial for memory. The use of antihistamines, either pharmaceutical or over the counter, is now reproducibly linked to an increased risk of cognitive decline and dementia, as well as to an increased risk of cancer and premature death. There are nineteen scientific investigations linking sleep hypnotics to premature death. This means that the link between taking sleeping pills and decreasing your time on earth is well established!

Downshifting to Gear Up

Thoughts Are Things

As we near the completion of this book, hopefully you have gained an appreciation for how much our brain is operating for us, what it's capable of, and all the things that can possibly cause it harm. As sensitive as our brain is to toxins, a lack of oxygen, and inflammation, we certainly don't want to burden our system more with unnecessary psychological stress, although we often do. We cannot always control what happens to us, but we can modify our response. This is what creates resilience. Resilience is a virtue that enables people to move through hardship and become better. Beliefs literally mold your brain.

In the section "Oxidative Stress and What Causes It" at the beginning of chapter 8, I mention a list of things that cause stress for the brain. At the end of that list are psychological stress and unresolved trauma. In this section, I will address some simple, practical ways to handle psychological stress, as well as some of the neuroscientific research behind it. Perceptions can please or paralyze your nervous system. Life's traumas and unwelcome experiences rewire and reorganize your brain's connections and communication systems in such a way as to make your response to life's stressors more rigid. With practice and effort these automatic nervous system responses can become more flexible.

In fact, a stiff, rigid, "hard" personality is reflective of stiff brain cells, rigid plaques that build up in the brain, and a general loss of resiliency. This is not a figurative metaphor. It is literally what happens in your brain. The exciting discovery of neuroplasticity is that our brain is constantly changing throughout life. Through different practices, we can sculpt healthy new pathways in the brain and prune away old ones, no matter how old we are!

Sculpting Our Brain

When we sculpt our brain to build in flexibility and memory, it thickens, quite literally. Building flexibility through meditation and memory by "working the brain" actually produces more neurons and more neural connections. This is often termed *synaptic density*. Each neuron has numerous arms that branch out to make connections with other neurons. These connections are only made when we encourage them to be made through the way we think and how often we think along the same pathway. That's why practice is required when you are trying to master a new skill—we need to do the same thing over and over again. Thickened parts of the brain on an MRI reveal where we have grown more neural tissue. A thickened brain is a smarter brain. Here is an excerpt from *Good Morning, I Love You* by Shauna Shapiro, PhD:

> *Research shows that London taxi drivers have bigger and stronger areas of the brain responsible for visual-spatial mapping and memory. Why does this happen? To operate one of London's iconic black taxi cabs in the complex urban maze of London's 25,000 streets, drivers must pass one of the most rigorous exams in the world, known simply as "the Knowledge." Drivers who pass the Knowledge study for an average of four years—that's as long as medical school in the US.*

Similarly, research by Sara Lazar, PhD, and her colleagues at Harvard used MRI to look at the brains of people who practice mindfulness. They found that the areas of the brain related to attention, learning, and emotional processing were bigger. Not only that, but "meditation practice may slow age-related thinning of the frontal cortex."[109]

One characteristic that is present in all healthy older people is resiliency—that hard-to-measure quality of adapting to change, shifting with changing tides rather than drowning, seeing the glass half full, or knowing how to turn lemons into lemonade. Our ability to be resilient is affected by our childhood and how we respond to our experiences. If we have had a blessed childhood with love, safety, and community, we tend to be more resilient. However, a childhood with stress and trauma can set us up for more challenges in our adult years.

The Stress and Relaxation Responses

The stress and relaxation responses are controlled by the brain's command and control center: the central autonomic nervous system. You actually have no control over your stress response. It is an autonomic function. That means it is not governed by conscious behavior. It happens automatically, the same as the circulation of your blood or the pumping of your heart. Any time you are exposed to something you perceive as stressful, your stress response is automatically switched on and you go into fight-or-flight mode.

During fight-or-flight, your adrenal glands are switched on, dumping excess cortisol, epinephrine (adrenaline), and norepinephrine (noradrenaline) into your bloodstream. Your heart begins to race, blood is shunned away from your brain to your legs, your eyes dilate, and you get ready to fight whatever is threatening you or to run like hell.

From an evolutionary perspective, this physiological response makes sense. Our ancestors needed these kinds of biochemical mechanisms if they were going to survive in the natural world. However, in our modern Western culture, few of us have to chase down animals for food or run from saber-toothed tigers. Yet this stress response still remains. Notice I said it gets triggered automatically by *anything* you perceive as stressful. This means that every time your boss scowls at you for being late, your kids spill milk on your lap at dinner, or your bank account is looking low, your stress response can get triggered. It doesn't stop there. Your stress response can also be initiated by these triggers:

A nutrient-depleted, toxic diet
Electropollution
Environmental toxins
Loss of control
Loss of community
Loss of a sense of purpose

This means that most of us are perpetually in a state of alarm. We never stop stressing out. Our bodies and brains were not designed to deal with all this chronic stress. In fact, unremitting stress literally eats away at the brain. Here are some of the negative effects it causes:

Damage to the hippocampus

Increased excitotoxicity, leading to cell death

Increased inflammation

Reduction in acetylcholine, affecting our memory

Reduction in serotonin levels, leading to anxiety and depression

Reduction in social interactions and sexual receptivity

There is an antidote to all this stress we experience. It is relaxation. You have some control over your relaxation response. Sitting on the sofa, channel surfing while sipping a glass of chardonnay, practicing retail therapy, or surfing the internet until late in the night can be helpful, but are limited. You have to consciously learn to relax. How do you do this?

Two Ways to Relax

There are two ways to relax:

1. Reduce stressful inputs in your life.
2. Learn to stimulate the part of your brain that helps you relax by developing a self-care program that you find easy and enjoyable to implement into your life.

Reduce Stressful Inputs by Identifying and Eliminating Stressors

Looking closely at the habits of our lives (both what we do and how we think) is not something most of us do on a regular basis. We often don't connect with how well we feel every day with the choices we make in our diet, in our relationships, in our work, or in the use of brain-altering substances like sugar, caffeine, and alcohol.

Eating junk food, drinking six cups of coffee a day, having one or two cocktails at night to calm down, watching four hours of television a day, doing work we hate, or being stuck in relationships that don't give us peace or joy are poor coping mechanisms. They add stress to our lives. They drive our mood and the functioning of our brain in the opposite direction from joy. They promote more of the brain chemicals that are detrimental and diminish the ones (such as serotonin) that help us to feel better.

Social or Psychological Stressors

Some examples of social and psychological stressors include these:

A challenging financial situation
An unsatisfactory job
Kids with challenging behaviors
Low self-confidence
Low self-esteem
Psychological disorders
Challenging relationships
The state of the world
Thoughts and beliefs about yourself that are negating

Physical Stressors

Some examples of physical stressors include these:

Alcohol, tobacco, and drugs
Allergens
Caffeine in high amounts

Chronic illness
Chronic infections
Overweight or obesity
Processed foods
Saturated trans fats
Sedentary lifestyle
Sugar and high-fructose corn syrup in the diet
Toxins

Life-Giving Activities

Some examples of life-giving activities include these:

Being in nature
Being with pets
Playing with grandchildren
Celebrations
Church or temple service, or devotional ritual
Community
Creative art, photography, or similar hobby
Dance
Exercise
Gardening
Intimate connection with a primary partner
Playing a musical instrument
Reading a novel
Sex
Shared healthy meals
Yoga classes

Stressors Versus Life-Giving Activities

Realistically, it is rare if not impossible that someone is able to eliminate all causes of stress in their life. We can, however, prevent unnecessary stressors or create healthy boundaries for ourselves. We can take an inventory—a close examination of our daily habits—to consider the things we can let go of that are triggering stress versus the things we can add that will help us to heal and thrive.

I suggest you do an exercise here to take a look at your own life. Take two different sheets of paper. On the first one, write your list of life-giving activities. On the second, write your list of stressors. Compare the length of your lists when you lay them side by side. Now, make an agreement with yourself to eliminate at least one thing this week that robs you of your energy and causes you stress. Add one thing to your life that gives you energy. Do this once a week and your life will transform.

Your weekly goals may look like this:

Do one thing I've always wanted to do but never done before (for me it was horseback riding along a wooded trail).

Invite a new friend over to dinner.

Make a collage of your dream home, vacation, or healthy body.

Play tennis with a friend.

Read the novel you've heard about.

Sleep in on a weekend morning.

Take a bubble bath one night this week.

Try playing a new instrument.

The Brain, Stress, and Our Childhood

Isn't it interesting that the same event or experience can have a different impact on different people? It would seem the determining factor is often the way we perceive our reality. Some people are more sensitive to stress due to their childhood or even birth trauma. A traumatic childhood can mold our reaction to stress negatively, making us more prone to illness and addictions. Emotional stressors growing up combined with severe trauma can affect the central nervous system. Our brains are more prone to the impact of traumatic events when we are young versus when we are older. The younger we are at the time of the trauma, the stronger the effect of the trauma on our nervous system. This is because the nervous system responds to the threat by upregulating our innate survival responses. The infant's or child's nervous system then becomes vigilant, on guard for a future repetition of the perceived threat (which could have been witnessing a violent fight between Mom and Dad or a sibling being hit by a parent). When a child observes a threatening event, defensive responses are activated. These responses look like fight, flight, or freeze and are mediated by the sympathetic nervous system and by the somatic nervous system and hypothalamic-pituitary-adrenal axis. Defensive responses can look like anger bursts that are impulsive, shallow breathing, high blood pressure, and anxiety. If a person has a healthy response, then when a threat is successfully negotiated and safety is re-established, defensive responses are downregulated and physiology returns to its homeostatic baseline.

The Adverse Childhood Experiences Study

The Adverse Childhood Experiences (ACEs) Study was conducted by the American Health Maintenance Organization, Kaiser Permanente, and the Centers for Disease Control and Prevention. Participants were recruited to the study between 1995 and 1997 and have been in long-term follow up for health outcomes. The study demonstrated an association of adverse childhood experiences (a.k.a. childhood trauma) with health and social problems across their lifespan, such as an increase in the total number of days lost from work as an adult. Felitti and Robert Anda from the

Centers for Disease Control and Prevention went on to survey childhood trauma experiences of over 17,000 Kaiser Permanente patient volunteers. The 17,337 participants were volunteers from approximately 26,000 consecutive Kaiser Permanente members. About half were female; 74.8 percent were white; the average age was 57; 75.2 percent had attended college; all had jobs and good health care, because they were members of the Kaiser health maintenance organization.

Participants were asked about ten types of childhood trauma that had been identified in earlier research literature:

Emotional abuse

Exposure to domestic violence

Household mental illness

Household substance abuse

Incarcerated household member

Parental separation or divorce

Physical abuse

Physical or emotional neglect

Sexual abuse

According to the US Substance Abuse and Mental Health Services Administration, the ACE study found that about two-thirds of individuals studied reported at least one adverse childhood experience; 87 percent of individuals who reported one ACE reported at least one additional ACE. The number of ACEs was strongly associated with adulthood high-risk health behaviors such as smoking, alcohol and drug abuse, and promiscuity, as well as with severe obesity, and correlated with ill-health, including depression, heart disease, cancer, chronic lung disease, and shortened lifespan. Compared to an ACE score of zero, having four adverse childhood experiences was associated with a seven-fold (700 percent) increase in alcoholism, a doubling of risk of being diagnosed with cancer, and a four-fold increase in emphysema; an ACE score above six was associated with a 30-fold (3000 percent) increase in attempted suicide.

The ACE study's results suggest that maltreatment and household dysfunction in childhood contribute to health problems decades later. The study was initially published in the *American Journal of Preventive Medicine*.[110] A self-assessment tool for ACE is in the resources section.

Addictions such as alcoholism are often our way of trying to cope with anxiety. There are healthier substances than alcohol that can assist a brain with anxiety. I like to support a person's nervous system with natural supplements for their brain health, which you can read about under the section "Calm Your Mind with Supplements" further along in this chapter.

Post-Traumatic Stress Disorder

Post-traumatic stress disorder (PTSD) is the most widely recognized trauma-related disorder and as such, serves as a good model for understanding the underlying processes involved in psycho-emotional trauma in general. The symptoms of PTSD include nightmares, unwanted memories of the trauma, avoidance of situations that bring back memories of the trauma, heightened reactions, hostility, agitation, irritability, hypervigilance, self-destructive behavior, and social isolation.

The excerpts below come from an article by Sandro D'Amico, ND, "Psycho-emotional Trauma: The Elephant in the Waiting Room," published in *Townsend Letter*, October 2016:

> *Studies have shown reduced volume of the orbitofrontal and medial prefrontal cortices in individuals with PTSD, as well as decreased blood flow to the medial prefrontal cortex in veterans with PTSD exposed to non-trauma-related stressful stimuli.... Lifetime prevalence of PTSD*

> *in American adults has been estimated at about 7%, although rates in specific types of traumatic exposure vary considerably.*
>
> *Studies of US veterans returning home from active duty in Iraq have reported rates between 4% and 17%. Approximately 9% of individuals involved in a motor vehicle accident subsequently develop PTSD.*
>
> *A large study of female sexual assault survivors found PTSD rates of 35.3% in those assaulted for the first time before age 18 and 30.2% for those first assaulted after age 18.*

The dominant psychotherapeutic approaches in use today for PTSD are cognitive behavioral therapy (CBT) and eye movement desensitization and reprocessing (EMDR). CBT, essentially talk therapy, has a very poor effectiveness based on research showing a nonresponse rate of up to 50 percent. While CBT and EMDR are certainly helpful, it is unclear to what degree they actually alter the physiological dysregulation underlying trauma.

Out of the need to treat trauma in a way that had not yet been attempted, several somatically based therapies have been developed. These include somatic experiencing, sensorimotor psychotherapy, and self-regulation therapy. These therapies currently lack validation by clinical trials. The common goal of these therapies is to assist the individuals to complete thwarted neurological and motor defense responses, which appear to remain encoded cortically and subcortically as part of the person's trauma-associated procedural memory. These therapies use mindful awareness of somatic sensations as a guide to identifying and completing defensive responses.

Self-regulation is one of the fundamental functions of the central nervous system and is essential for long-term health. Through self-regulation and self-soothing practices, a person with PTSD can begin to bring their neurotransmitters, hormones, and hypothalamus, pituitary gland, and adrenal glands axis back into alignment.

Part of caring for the healing of a traumatized brain will require a person to assess their home and work environments for how supportive they are. It is necessary to try to create an environment that is healing and free of social stressors such as those named above. If a person had these stressors as a child growing up, their nervous system has a different reaction to stress than someone who did not grow up with these stressors.

Somatic-based self-regulation encourages you to maintain an aware connection with your body, realizing that the mind is in sympathy with the body and that bodily composure facilitates mental clarity and calmness.

Eleven Minutes to Inner Peace

Pause and try a somatic-based self-regulation exercise.

First, take one minute to stop reading, place one hand on your chest and one on your belly, and sense your body. Tune in. If you could come up with a word for a sensation you are feeling in your body, what would it be? *Tight jaw, cold feet,* or *warm hands*, for example. Think of a feeling state also; it may be *curious*, *bored*, or *inspired.*

Next, spend ten minutes doing a different activity, such as soft belly breathing, described later in this chapter. Now go back to tuning in by placing one hand on your heart and the other on your belly. Is there a word to describe what you're sensing, and is there a word for your emotion? Has your bodily sensation or emotional sensation changed after completing the breathing exercise?

Dealing with Feelings

We are born into this world in baby bodies that are usually free of disease. We smile and coo naturally; our minds are awake and playful.

Yet sometimes even when we are in our mother's womb and after our birth, life begins to unravel as its own unique set of circumstances. These circumstances begin to mold our attitudes, life viewpoints, biases, proclivities, and brains. If we are lucky, we have a safe and stable source of shelter and food. Our personalities, however, have basic existential needs that go far beyond food and shelter. In fact, these needs are outlined by Marshall Rosenberg in his body of work called "nonviolent communication" and published in his book of the same name. In this body of work, Rosenberg states that all human beings have basic elemental needs. It is very rare that we have all these needs fulfilled at one point in time, but they are core essential needs.

Taking an inventory of these needs is a valuable exercise, as once we realize they exist, we can bring more of them into our lives. Here are lists of these personality needs:

Autonomy

Choice, freedom, independence, space, spontaneity

Connection

Acceptance, affection, appreciation, belonging, cooperation, communication, closeness, community, companionship, compassion, consideration, consistency, empathy, inclusion, intimacy, love, mutuality, nurturing, respect/self-respect, safety, security, stability, support, to know and be known, to see and be seen, to understand and be understood, trust, warmth

Honesty

Authenticity, integrity, presence

Meaning

Awareness, celebration of life, challenge, clarity, competence, consciousness, contribution, creativity, discovery, efficacy, effectiveness, growth, hope, learning, mourning, participation, purpose, self-expression, stimulation, to matter, understanding

Peace

Beauty, communion, ease, equality, harmony, inspiration, order

Physical Well-Being

Air, food, movement and exercise, rest and sleep, sexual expression, safety, shelter, touch, water

Play

Joy, humor, non-goal-oriented activity that brings laughter or a sense of fun

Depending on your psychological state, simply reading this list of needs may make you feel inwardly sad or alarmed that you have so many that are unmet. That's how I felt when I first read them. Alternatively, you may feel really good in this area. This would mean that your social, family, and community lifestyles are supportive.

The field of psychoneuroimmunology studies the connections between our minds and bodies. It has shown through its research that our immune systems and brains are wired together through an elaborate communication system. Not having our needs met can lead to anger and other emotions such as shame, frustration, grief, or numbing out. Anger, both expressed or ignored, will trigger the amygdala in the brainstem, which then signals the hypothalamus. The hypothalamus releases corticotropin-releasing hormone to the pituitary gland. The pituitary sends a message to the adrenals via adrenocorticotropic-releasing hormones, triggering the release of adrenalin, cortisol, and norepinephrine, the stress hormones.

Long-term stress hormones produced by anger or suppressed anger, or by other strong toxic emotions, can negatively impact our microbial diversity, immune function, hormone balance, thyroid functioning, and cardiovascular function, and can cause inflammation.

In her article in the *Psychological Bulletin*, "Stress, Emotion, and Human Immune Function," Ann O'Leary, PhD, highlights a study in which individuals who disclosed a tragic event seemed to have an elevated immune response and generally were healthier than those who inhibited expression of those emotions.[111] The field of psycho-immunology studies this link between our emotional world and our immune system and its link with different disease states.

Here are some ways to proactively navigate your feelings:

Be honest with yourself, get in touch with your core feelings around a situation. For example, maybe you realize you were actually jealous of the attention an older sibling got.

Choose forgiveness. Forgiveness is extremely powerful. One study by Fred Luskin, PhD, involved a forgiveness process that mothers whose children had been murdered underwent; this involvement greatly improved their emotional state. In his book *Forgive for Good,* Dr. Luskin offers a groundbreaking study based on scientific research from the frontiers of psychology and medicine.

Discharge your feelings. Some emotions can be very strong and highly charged. Simply being aware of our feelings often doesn't allow the associated energetic charge to be released. When discharging an emotion, you don't want to aim that charge at the other person. If you are angry, for example, you don't want to scream at the other person. Instead, use a sport such as tennis, racquetball, or volleyball to vent your pent-up energy. Dig a ditch with a spade and funnel your energetic charge into the physical movement. Channel your frustration into shoving the spade into the ground and throwing the soil over your back. Take a pillow and punch it when no one is around or scream into it. Channel that energy by going running. Think of what it is you're angry about and place that energy in your legs, letting them push against the ground as you run. You can also take a kick-boxing class or a martial arts class like karate or judo. If you are unable to be physically active, then journaling or painting your feelings and the charge you have on a situation can be very helpful alternatives.

Get closer to your feelings and **choose courage**. This can be scary, but moving through your feelings with journaling, movement, and even tears can be incredibly cathartic and healing.

Get help by learning an effective form of therapy or nonviolent communication to communicate your feelings. You may not be able to resolve the issue with the person who is making you feel a certain way, but you can express your feelings to a healthy surrogate, such as a therapist, church minister, synagogue practitioner, or close friend.

Look at the role models you grew up with around anger. Did your parents deal with their feelings by numbing out in addiction, ignoring them, dismissing them, eating comfort food, being workaholics, imploding inwardly, or committing acts of self-harm? Realize that you may need to unlearn the behaviors that you automatically mirror from your parents. These behaviors are often deeply patterned into our way of being and we often have blind spots to them. Usually it's our marital partner or a person we live with or are closest to who can give us honest reflection about our toxic behaviors. We cannot change what we are unwilling to be aware of. Asking for honest feedback from a person close to you is a courageous act that has rich results.

Cultivating a Sense of Well-Being

I would like to take a moment here to highlight two key feeling states that can help one cultivate a sense of well-being: joy and faith. True joy is the depth of each moment; it is a sense of connectedness and presence of heart. One can feel deep joy just sitting in a chair, looking out a window and watching a tree, or smelling a flower. Joy comes on the wings of a sense of deep sincerity for the nature and beauty of something that exists, such as our furry pets that wag their tails in excitement when they see us or the grateful feedback of our loved ones when they eat a meal we've made for them. Our sense of well-being also comes from a sense of caring for others and being cared for ourselves. These things bring true joy. Joy, in and of itself, is a form of medicine.

Faith is knowing and trusting that goodness is held for us: a good life, resilient energy for the day, pleasure for our bodies, respite for our fatigue, wealth for our senses, solidity for our homes, and a future that is better than the one that was stolen from us by poor health. Having faith forms a bedrock that can support us through challenging times.

Sometimes you may feel far from faith and joy. You may feel trapped in a place of victimhood, stress, compression, fear, and isolation. If you are feeling far from joy, you may need help to reconnect with your faith. You may choose to reach out to your pastor at church or a rabbi at your nearest temple or an interfaith ministry in your town to help you build a sense of divine support and community. Some people do not resonate with any kind of religion or faith; you may want to explore this area in your life. Consider reading the book *A Course in Miracles* or *The Way of Grace: The Transforming Power of Ego Relaxation* by Miranda Macpherson.

Calm Your Mind with Herbal Medicine

You can reduce the overactivity and increase the resilience of your nervous system by using adaptogenic herbs (named because they may help you adapt to stress). Much like culinary spices, herbs were meant by Mother Nature to be taken in combination. The adaptogenic herbs I use are in formulas that mix several herbs together. Adaptogens include these supplements, many of which I mentioned in chapter 4:

Ashwagandha

Holy basil

Rhodiola root extract

St. John's wort

Learning to Push the Pause Button

The real key to eliminating stress is learning to relax. My favorite ways to do this are these:

Connecting socially and being with loved ones

Meditating

Soft belly breathing

Let's talk about each of these.

Connecting Socially and Being with Loved Ones

Having supportive and encouraging people in your life makes a huge difference in being able to move forward toward being our best selves. Take the time every day to connect with friends and family. Connecting over dinner has been shown to actually increase the IQ of children! Having a "date night" to have fun with your significant other is also important. In fact, the act of play produces a brain chemical that goes along the same track as trauma in the brain. Play heals trauma. Find exercise that is *fun* for you. Laughter is healing too. In fact, there is an entire branch of yoga called laughter yoga. Invest in positive relationships throughout your life but especially while trying to recuperate from a health challenge. Consider a life coach to help you if there's no one in your life right now. Or join a support group, church, or synagogue.

Meditating

Among its many benefits, meditating reduces stress. Think of your brain as a computer that is simultaneously keeping many windows open and many programs going. Meditating helps you close the unnecessary windows so you can focus on what's essential. **When you do less with more, you enjoy life more and perform at a higher level.** The positive effects of meditation are astounding and certainly deserve your contemplation and consideration if you're not already a consistent meditator. Many successful businesspeople, celebrities, and sports professionals practice regularly and enjoy the positive effects of meditation. Research has scientifically proven that meditation is a safe and simple way to balance your physical, emotional, and mental states, and more and more doctors are encouraging patients to practice meditation to cure many stress-related illnesses.

Still, I know meditation is not easy for everyone, which is why I encourage you to find a practice that works for you. Here are some of my favorite resources:

> Smartphone app: Mindrise: Sleep & Meditation. You can find my meditations when you sign up and go to the "meditations" tab; I am listed as one of the teachers.
>
> In-person classes and retreats:
>
> Spirit Rock in Woodacre, CA
>
> The Center in San Francisco
>
> Esalen Institute in Big Sur, CA
>
> 1440 Multiversity in California

Anchor Meditation in San Francisco

The Monkhouse Method Yoga

Laughter Yoga

Soft Belly Breathing

The following excerpt is from *Clarity and Calm: An Everyday Guide to Mindfulness* by Buddhist monk and author Ajahn Sucitto. As you read it, do the actual practice at the same time.

> *Spend some time establishing the breathing as a flow. Find a place where you can be seated with your spine straight, but relaxed. This may mean getting some pillows behind your back. Drop your shoulders, relax your face and center your breathing in the abdomen. Gently breathe out completely, then wait for the in-breath; let your breathing naturally lengthen and deepen.*
>
> *Feel the energy in the flow of breathing. This is not confined to a particular point, though you might want to rest your attention at a place in your belly, diaphragm, chest or nostrils and sense the breathing flowing through it. When you breathe in, can you feel a sense of brightening? With the outbreath, do you get a sense of releasing? The sense is not of air, but of a changing energy, right? Let your body fully feel that flow as it causes it to swell and subside in a regular way. Through this process, your body-energy gathers within the breathing. Whatever you're currently feeling in terms of bodily vitality or nervous energy, bring that to the breathing. So, this means if you feel tired, dull or stagnant—or if you feel speedy or agitated—breathe into that. Don't struggle with the tiredness but also don't sink into it. Don't try to shut down the speediness but don't add to it with distracting actions. Instead, "hold" these energies, just as energies within the breathing. Let your breathing be long and deep and bring the current state of bodily energy into contact with its flow. Open to your bodily experience and let your breath-flow inhabit it. It's rather like putting on a new suit and getting comfortable in it. Feel what it's like for awareness to spread over, include and know your body and its energy.*[112]

Alternatively, you can search on Pandora.com or Spotify.com for Karen Drucker's song "Breathe." While you listen, sit with your spine straight and supported. Alternatively, download the iPhone app Mindrise and choose a five- to ten-minute meditation to relax along with.

10 BUILDING NEW NEURAL PATHWAYS

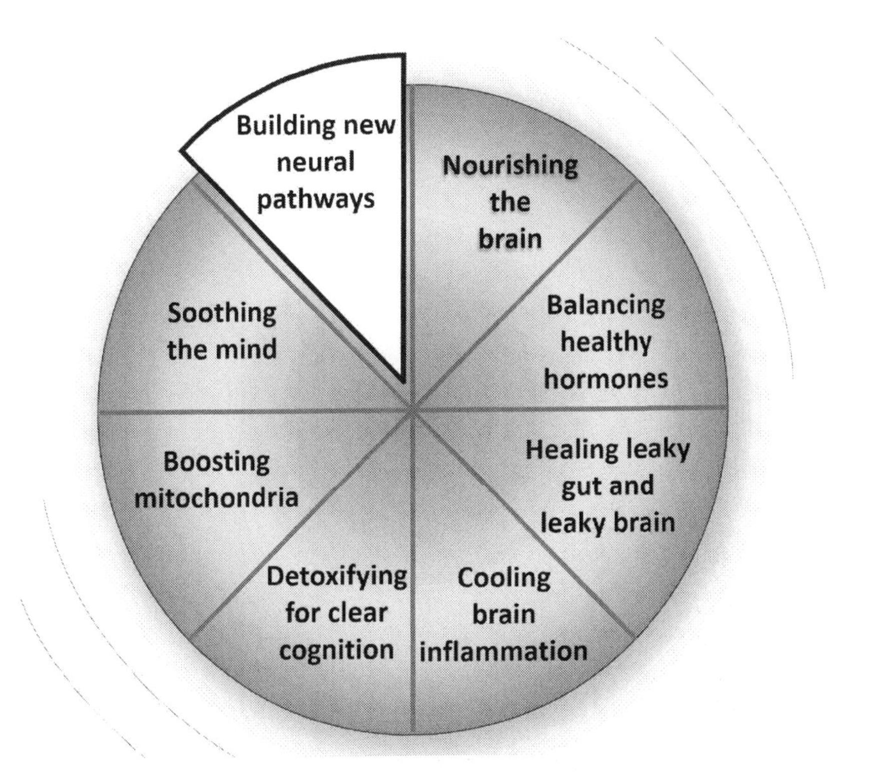

An often ignored yet important aspect of our anatomy is that we are electromagnetic beings. This is why it's possible to get an electrocardiogram (ECG) reading from electrodes placed on a person's chest to measure heart rate variability, and an electroencephalogram (EEG) reading from electrodes placed on a person's skull to measure brain waves. Perhaps the most common examples of modern medicine's intersection with the electrical aspect of our physical body is in the instances of an ECG being used in the emergency department of a hospital to find evidence of a heart attack and an EEG being used on the head to find evidence of seizure activity.

What's even more fascinating is that our electrical nature goes deeper than the measurement of these two organs (the heart and the brain): it can be found in each cell. Each of our individual cells carries an electrical charge. For example, a healthy cell has an electrical potential of 90 mV (90 millivolts), an inflamed cell measures 120 mV, and a degenerating cell 30 mV.

In the 1960s German physicist Fritz-Albert Popp discovered that cancer cells have a common feature of scrambling light in a chaotic way. From a medical point of view, we as living organisms can now be thought of as holographic wave patterns of photonic light energy. Recent research is showing that biophotons (ultraweak photon emissions) are released by all biological systems. These electromagnetic waves are in the optical frequency range, meaning that they manifest as light. Prior to the manifestation of a disease state, photonic light loses its rhythm as a harmonized flow of energy in the body. Reestablishing this rhythm brings your body back into its highest vibrational alignment, emotionally, mentally, physically, and spiritually.

When we understand ourselves as electromagnetic beings, we begin to open the door to the regenerative properties of the energy that is shifting and moving throughout our body. The classical model of Chinese medicine and the ancient yogic practices of India have understood this for thousands of years. In fact, numerous studies show that yoga reduces symptoms of depression and anxiety in older women, compared with controls.[113]

Biological electricity is the phenomenon arising from movements of the charged ions (such as sodium, potassium, chloride, calcium, and magnesium) across the cell membranes in our body. Nerve conduction relies on these electrochemical processes; electricity arises because of the difference in electrical polarity from one side of our cell membranes to the other. Depolarization and repolarization of cell membranes allow nerves to conduct signals from place to place in the body.

The entire living matrix of a human body is simultaneously a mechanical, vibrational, energetic, electronic, and informational network.

Our Biofield and Coherence as a Factor of Healing

The collective energy generated by the body and mind can be referred to as a *biofield*. The biofield is described in terms of three fundamental energies enfolded within each other: quantum fields, potential fields, and classical electromagnetic fields (EMFs). It is constantly changing and reflects a totality of our body's coherent light production and therefore wholeness.

This is an excerpt from Peter Fraser and Harry Massey's book *Decoding the Human Body-Field*, from the chapter "The Microworld and the Macroworld":

> *To study a cell, biologists dissolve it in a solution or grind it and then separate out its constituent parts, destroying the cell in order to study it. This is reductionist science at its best. It works beautifully. By taking apart cells, biologists learned that they have a complex and intricate structure. However, this is not* integrative *science. As cell biologist Franklin M. Harold wrote, "We know in our hearts that a cell is far more than an aggregate of individual molecules; it is an organized, structured, purposeful and evolved whole. Unfortunately, analytical practice dictates that we begin our inquiries by grinding the exquisite architecture of the living cell into a pulp. No wonder, then, that the integrative perspective is woefully absent from the molecular view of life as it has developed over the past half-century!" Integrative science strives to understand the whole in which emergent properties express themselves and so reveal functions and processes that are undecipherable*

> *and undetectable at lower levels. Integrative science is about connections at the systems level, about patterns that are revealed holistically and about simplicities that arise from a cluster of complexities. It is a science of synthesis.*

Taking a broader view, we are not just a mechanistic bag of molecules and organs bouncing against each other to form either health or disease. We are also emotional, sensitive, intuitive, perceptive, interpretive, and rational beings. In fact, our emotions, feelings, and thoughts make up most of our experience of the world.

Coherence as a Factor for Healing

This is an excerpt from chapter 3 of Peter Fraser and Harry Massey's book *Decoding the Human Body-Field*:

> *A team led by Korean scientists confirmed what other researchers in Germany, Japan, Russia, Poland, Italy, China and the United States have found—that the body does indeed emit ultraweak coherent light. In their article "Biophoton Emission from the Hands," the Korean-led team reported that they detected 34 percent more biophotons (in the range of 300–650 nanometers) coming from the hands of their twenty healthy volunteers than could be expected if the photons were simply a result of natural background emissions. They also confirmed that the biophotons were not created as a consequence of thermal radiation or body heat.... Fritz Popp found coherent light in the body. This amounted to an overturning of some of the most deeply entrenched beliefs in physics and biology. What's so special about coherent light? Well, it means that individual photons somehow become connected and cooperative, working together to transmit information about the state of the system. Think of an unruly crowd of fans at a football game suddenly focusing their attention and rising together in groups to do the wave cheer. That's*

coherence at work. The individuals are still individuals, but for a certain amount of time they come together, acting as one, in a purposeful behavior that has meaning.

Coherence is at least partly within our control. Studies have shown that holding positive thoughts in our heart creates coherence between electric and biophoton emissions, which then changes our DNA so that our body becomes healthier. In other words, DNA can at least partly be controlled by our thoughts.

Concerns about Cell Phone Towers, Smart Meters, and Wi-Fi

Now that you understand the crucial aspect of our anatomy known as the biofield, which embraces our electromagnetic nature as a core part of our health, we can begin to wonder whether the EMFs that cell phone towers, smart meters, and Wi-Fi generate are also potential toxins. When we think of toxins we normally think of chemicals, but this concern refers to the EMFs that can interfere with our physiological processes.

EMFs Can Cause Addiction and Changes in the Brain

Technology fulfills our need for stimulation, instant gratification, rapid change in environment, and connection with others. We need to be careful, though, as it can stimulate the brain in the same way an addictive substance does, and it can eventually be more appealing than real contact and intimacy, more appealing than actual relating or being in nature itself.

In a study that involved over 1,500 professionals throughout the US and Europe, research found that 40.2 percent considered proximity to Wi-Fi their first priority for luxury or necessity, followed by sex at 36.6 percent and alcohol at 14.3 percent. In fact, physicians may soon need to come up with the diagnosis of internet addiction disorder or gaming disorder, which is under debate in Japan right now as a possible new disorder classification for the ICD-11. A fascinating study published January 11, 2012, entitled "Abnormal White Matter Integrity in Adolescents with Internet Addiction Disorder: A Tract-Based Spatial Statistics Study" showed there were actual changes in the white matter functioning of the brains in those with internet addiction syndrome.[114]

The 2015 International EMF Scientist Appeal, signed by more than 230 scientists, called for the UN Environment Program to "investigate the potential for harm being posed to plants, animals and humans by man-made, non-ionizing electromagnetic field (EMF) pollution." These scientists have published peer-reviewed research on EMFs' influence on human biology and health and are calling for the strengthening of EMF guidelines and regulatory standards. These experts reported "serious concerns" regarding the ubiquitous and increasing exposure to EMFs. Their appeal refers to numerous scientific publications that show that EMFs "affect living organisms at levels well below most international and national guidelines." These effects include increased risks of cancer, neurological disorders, and reproductive harm.[115]

The Body Electric and Therapeutic Technology

Paracelsus said, "The dose makes the poison." In other words, a substance—in this case, the electromagnetic field—can be a medicine or a poison depending on the dosage.

There are two pieces of technology among probably a hundred or so that I would like to touch upon in my book: pulsed electromagnetic field (PEMF) therapy devices and mindfulness smartphone apps.

A Pulsed Electromagnetic Field Therapy Device

The vascular therapy mat is a patented PEMF device that I have been introduced to, and I have been impressed by its ability to increase oxygenation and microcirculation by up to 30 percent. In our body we have 70,000 miles of capillaries, tiny blood vessels that are one-sixth the size of a strand of hair, or less than 100 microns. If we laid out our capillaries in single file, they would wrap around the world three times! In these capillaries, which make up our microcirculation, oxygen is delivered from red blood cells into the tissues. Therefore, increasing circulation in the capillary has a powerful effect on the delivery of oxygen to the tissue. The vascular therapy mat helps by ensuring optimized microcirculation. Optimizing circulation in this way guarantees that each individual cell is supplied with the required oxygen and nutrients while removing metabolic waste. The device uses a patented wave form of the next generation of PEMF devices, which enables the body to work towards balancing *all* systems. It enhances vasomotion, which is the blood vessel's tone. Through vasomotion, the blood vessel constricts or oscillates spontaneously to move blood or venous fluid forward, independent of heartbeat, innervation, or respiration.

Here are the benefits of this device:

- Boosts the immune system
- Helps the cells function more efficiently
- Improves vasomotion of the microcirculation
- Improves immune response
- Enhances wound healing
- Increases oxygenation of tissues up to 30 percent
- Increases ATP production by 18 percent for 24 hours
- Improves nutrient delivery to the cells
- Improves waste disposal from the cells
- Enhances cardiac function
- Improves physical fitness, endurance, strength, and energy level
- Improves mental acuity, concentration, and focus

The device is a mat which a person lies on for eight minutes, optimally twice a day. It has a specific signal that supports enhanced vasomotion. The effect of this electromagnetic field on the rhythmic change in the diameter of arterioles and small arteries plays a vital role in the distribution of blood throughout the tissues.

Pierluigi Pompei of the University of Camerino, Italy, said in a 2017 presentation:

> *Electromagnetic field therapy has been used in healing for decades and has been reported to be beneficial in patients with a variety of diseases. A particular system is the patented PEMF mat, a Physical Vascular Therapy for which a normalization of the microcirculation has been demonstrated by a low frequency, pulse electromagnetic field pattern. This therapy, with a series of half-wave-shaped sinusoidal intensity variations was shown to increase vasomotion and microcirculation for improved organ blood flow, supply of nutrients, and removal of metabolites. Aim of our study was to evaluate the effects of this PEMF device on patients with cognitive deficits (dementia) and to subsequently monitor cognitive and genetic testing. A limited number of subjects (15 patients), ranging from 80–95 years old were recruited from the Ceci retirement home of Camerano, Italy. Physical Vascular Therapy treatment was given three times a week on recruited patients for eight consecutive weeks. In order to evaluate the Resistive and Pulsatility Index, using a Mindray transcranial doppler via a 2 MHx probe, median cerebral arterial prior and after BEMER treatment were monitored. Blood samples to evaluate oxidative stress through the paraoxonase enzyme, salivary swab testing for determination the APOE4 allele which has been shown to be associated with an increased risk of the AD and cognitive test were also recorded. As results from the cognitive test, we found 60% improvement in cognitive ability and perception of space and time. Taken together these findings show that BEMER therapy may therefore contribute to an ameliorated cerebral blood flow that could be an important factor involving in AD, thus clearly improving the quality of life.*[116]

To learn more about these devices, please contact Health and Wellness Navigator Linda Hetzel at 415-328-5060 or at Linda@LindaHetzel.com.[117]

Mindfulness Smartphone Apps

The second piece of technology I'd like to mention here is the Mindrise iPhone app *Sleep, Meditation, Music & Astrology.* Meditation aims to cultivate increased moment-to-moment awareness of one's thoughts, feelings, and bodily sensations while maintaining an open mind free from distraction and judgement. Naturopathic physician Krista Anderson-Ross published an article titled "We Are What We Think: Downregulating the Chronic Stress Response with Technology-Assisted Mindfulness Meditation" in the *Journal of Restorative Medicine* (2019; 8: page 3):

> *Meditation has been shown to produce positive effects on psychological well-being that extend beyond the time the individual is formally meditating, leading to decreased physiological markers of stress in a range of populations. A 2017 meta-analysis of 45 studies concluded that when all meditation subtypes were analyzed together, meditation reduced cortisol, C-reactive protein, blood pressure, heart rate, triglycerides and tumor necrosis factor-alpha. In other studies on the effects of mindfulness, concentration, attention, serenity, and ability to tolerate negative emotions have been shown to increase.*[118]

A study of 238 participants used a smartphone app to investigate whether a mindfulness meditation program could improve psychological well-being, reduce job strain, and reduce ambulatory blood pressure during the workday in middle-aged adults. Participants were asked to complete one 10- to 20-minute guided audio meditation per day for eight weeks. Psychosocial measures and blood pressure throughout one working day were measured, once at baseline and again eight weeks later. As well, a follow-up survey was completed sixteen weeks after the start of the intervention. Compared with control subjects, the intervention group reported significant improvement in global well-being; daily positive affect, anxiety and depressive symptoms; job strain; and workplace social support. These were sustained at eight weeks and sixteen weeks. In addition, a marginally significant decrease in self-measured systolic blood pressure from before to after intervention was noted. The researchers concluded that short guided mindfulness meditation delivered via smartphone and practiced multiple times per week can improve outcomes related to work stress and well-being, with potentially lasting effects.[119]

More Ways to Support Balance in Your Life

Journaling and body-based therapies are two of my favorite ways to balance the sea of emotions that can arise with the stresses of life. They simply allow me to catch up with my own self, slow down, and delight in the moment.

Journal to Music

Journaling to music can be particularly evocative. Music to journal by includes the music of Olafur Arnalds, Kristin Hoffman, Sacred Earth, Deuter, R. Carlos Nakai, Steven Halpern, and Gary Malkin.

Here is a list of questions you can reflect upon and write about in your journal while you listen to some of this music:

> How would you live if you knew that you were going to die in one year?
>
> Name five things that you do for yourself.
>
> List five things that you prefer to do alone.
>
> List five things that you prefer to do with others.
>
> Describe yourself using five different words.
>
> What would you say is your most important achievement so far?
>
> If you had only three days left to live, what would you do?
>
> What do you feel are your limitations?
>
> Can you call this a good life?

Fill in: I'm afraid of ...

Fill in: I'm angry about ...

Fill in: I'm grateful for ...

Fill in: I need ...

What's working in your life right now?

What's not working in your life right now?

If your future healthy self, ten years from now, could give you a message that would bring you toward your own best self and best life, what would it be?

If there is one thing that would make the biggest difference in your life right now, what would it be?

If you could change one thing about yourself, what would it be?

If journaling is new to you, one place you can start is to write down five things about your day that you are grateful for; you can do this each night before you go to bed. Shawn Achor, a Harvard graduate, wrote a book called *The Happiness Advantage* after doing a research study showing that no matter our age, bringing grateful awareness to a few things each day actually changes our brains to help us achieve more joy in our lives!

Our body holds cellular memories in its tissues. Sometimes we unconsciously store emotions as tension in our body. Therefore, body-based therapies such as yoga, massage, biofeedback, dance, chanting, qigong, and dynamic meditation can bring a flow of energy to these areas and release stored tension.

Try This Five-Minute Somatic-Based Awareness Exercise

A somatic-based awareness exercise is an exercise to help you find a way to connect with your body. Our body is not meant to be split and fragmented into parts. We are not walking brains on a stick. When we connect to self with awareness in a slow, subtle way we are engaging the principles of neuroplasticity that allow for new neural circuitry. This involves movement in which the focus is not goal oriented, as in contractions for muscle tone building, but rather a gentle awareness in a slow way and with freedom for variation. Including visualization and imagination with the movement aids in laying down new neural pathways. The brain loves to learn new things and it responds to a fresh outlook.

Instructions

Find a quiet place where you are undisturbed for one minute. Find a place where you can be seated with your spine straight but relaxed. This may mean getting some pillows behind your back. Drop your shoulders and relax your face. Imagine a bright yellow sun the size of a tennis ball at the base of your skull and top of your neck, just where the skull sits upon your neck, like a golf ball on a tee. Very slowly, at the pace of a sunset, flex your chin toward your chest and place the tip of your tongue behind your front teeth, resting it gently there. Then slowly bring your head back up to neutral. Now imagine that you have a blue sky the size of a tennis ball and place that again at the same place at the top of your neck. At the same slow pace as before, extend your head up toward the ceiling and then back to neutral.

Pause and notice if there are any changes in how you feel. Are your thoughts quieter, for example? Did you perhaps feel a pulsing in your hands or feet?

Try it again, but this time use the blue-sky image when you flex your chin forward and then the bright yellow sun when you extend your head. Is there one version that feels more balancing to you than the other? Consider playing some music while you do this, such as Steven Halpern's "Om Zone 2.0"

Time Away

Sometimes it helps to detach from everything and go away for a week or a long weekend retreat in nature or in beauty.

Pet Therapy

Many of us can resonate with the saying that a dog is man's best friend. Personally, I'm a cat lover, and my feline friends were some of the closest to my heart when I was a little girl growing up. No one else could climb up onto my chest and purr itself to sleep when I lived in a household of adversity as a young girl. Sometimes our pets give us a sense of unconditional love that no human ever can. After the death of a family member later in my life, I became a horse owner. The stunning beauty and sensitivity of my horse challenges me to be a better person with a deeper quality of presence. Be open to having a close relationship with a pet.[120]

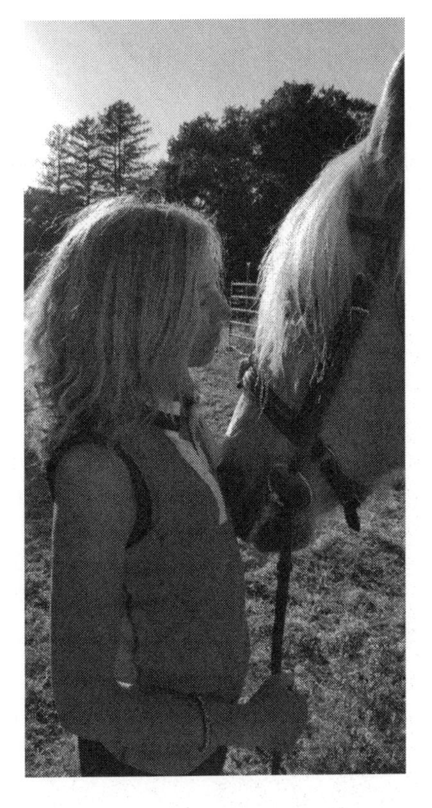

Forest Bathing

Part of my family roots are German. When in Germany, you do as the Germans do, which frequently involves getting together and taking a day long hike in the woods on a Sunday. Recently, Japan actually created the term *forest bathing*, based on research showing that the woods have healing properties. There is a whole new type of healing modality based on forest bathing.[121]

PART THREE

Life's traumas and unwelcome experiences rewire and reorganize your brain's connections and make your response to life more rigid. With practice and effort these responses can become more flexible.

—Dr. Jacqueline Chan

RESOURCES

Dietary fiber is plant material that is an essential element in optimal gut health. It is normally left undigested after passing through the body's digestive system. Food sources of dietary fiber are often classified according to whether they contain predominantly *soluble* or *insoluble* fiber. Plant foods usually contain a combination of both types of fiber in varying degrees, according to the plant's characteristics.

Insoluble Fiber

Insoluble fiber, found in certain plant foods, particularly whole grains, absorbs water throughout the digestive system, helping to promote regular, healthy bowel movements by binding with water and forming a gel. This allows the body's waste to form into soft and bulky stools, which helps to efficiently rid the body of toxins. Wheat bran is a good source of insoluble fiber. While we cannot digest the insoluble fiber in wheat bran, it is partially digested by beneficial bacteria in the gut, helping to ferment them into short-chain fatty acids that nourish our intestines.

Soluble fiber

Soluble fiber, found in all plant foods, dissolves in water to form a gel-like substance. It is readily fermented in the colon and includes other plant components such as lignans, oligosaccharides, polysaccharides, resistant starches, and inulin. Soluble fiber also promotes soft and bulky stools, delays gastric emptying, and binds with bile acids, helping to lower cholesterol levels. Foods that are considered good sources of soluble fiber include oat bran, guar gum, dried beans and peas, apples with skin, seaweeds, and flaxseeds.

- **Lignans**, a soluble fiber found in flaxseeds, wheat, and legumes, are known to possess anticancer, antibacterial, and antiviral properties. They bind to estrogen receptors in the body, interfering with cancer promotion and helping to regulate estrogen levels. Soluble fiber also promotes a delay in the absorption of glucose and increases insulin sensitivity, resulting in improved glucose metabolism, ultimately helping to lower the risk of type 2 diabetes.
- **Inulin** is another soluble fiber that is not digested in the upper gastrointestinal tract. Low in calories, inulin stimulates the growth of beneficial bacteria, and does not lead to a rise in serum glucose or stimulate insulin secretion. Inulin has been used to improve the taste of low-fat foods. Fructo-oligosaccharides (FOS) are the most common example of inulin. FOS have a sweet, pleasant flavor and can be used to fortify foods with fiber, to improve the flavor of low-calorie foods, and to improve the texture of lower-fat foods. Because these fibers stimulate the growth of beneficial bacteria, they are also called prebiotics. Besides FOS, good sources of inulin include artichokes, garlic, leeks, onions, chicory, tofu and other soy products, and grains such as barley, flax, oat, and wheat.

Grams of Fiber in Foods

All fruits and vegetables contain fiber, but some have more than others. The list below focuses on the more important fiber sources. If there are less than 2 g of fiber in a typical serving of a fruit or vegetable, it is not listed. At least 20–35 g of fiber is suggested each day by the American Dietetic Association.

Beans

Amy's Black Bean Chili, 1 cup: 13.0 g

Amy's Indian Palak Paneer, 1 container (frozen): 6.0 g

Black beans, ½ cup cooked: 7.5 g

Edamame, ½ cup cooked: 3.8 g

Gardenburger, 1 patty (fiber depends on variety chosen): 4.0–5.0 g

Green peas, ½ cup cooked: 3.7 g

Health Valley Minestrone Soup, 1 cup: 7.0 g

Health Valley Vegetarian Santa Fe White Bean Chili, 1 cup: 9.0 g

Hummus, ¼ cup: 3.7 g

Kidney beans, ½ cup cooked: 6.6 g

Lentils, ½ cup cooked: 7.8 g

Lima beans, ½ cup cooked: 6.6 g

Nile Spice Lentil Soup (dehydrated), 1 container: 11.0 g

Pinto beans, ½ cup cooked: 5.5 g

Progresso 3 Bean Chili with Beef, 1 cup: 7.0 g

Progresso Lentil Soup, 1 cup: 5.0 g

Split peas, ½ cup cooked: 8.0 g

Breads

Ezekiel Sprouted Whole Grain Breads, 1 slice: 3.0 g

Ezekiel Sprouted Whole Grain Tortillas, 1: 5.0 g

Great Harvest Caraway Rye, 1 slice: 5.0 g

High Fiber Bread, 1 slice: 6.0 g

La Tortilla Factory Smart and Delicious High Fiber Tortillas, 1: 12.0 g

La Tortilla Factory Smart and Delicious Whole Wheat Tortillas, 1: 8.0 g

Mission Carb Balance Whole Wheat or plain Whole Wheat Tortillas, 1: 8.0 g

Cereals

Arrowhead Mills Bran Flakes, 1 cup: 4.0 g

Barbara's Breakfast O's, 1¼ cups: 3.0 g

Kashi 7 Whole Grain Nuggets, ½ cup: 7.0 g

Kashi 7 Whole Grain Pilaf, ½ cup: 6.0 g

Post Grape Nuts, ½ cup: 7.0 g

Post Shredded Wheat, 2 biscuits: 6.0 g

Quaker Oat Bran Cereal, ½ cup cooked: 6.0 g

Wheatena, 1 cup cooked: 7.0 g

Crackers, Seeds, and Nuts

Chia seeds, 1 tbsp.: 6.8 g

Coconut (unsweetened), 3 tbsp. grated: 2.4 g

Coconut flour, 2 tbsp.: 6.0 g

Flaxseed, 2 tbsp. ground: 4.0 g

Lundberg Organic Sesame Tamari Rice Cakes, 1: 2.0 g

Ryvita Sesame Rye or Pumpkin Seeds and Oats, 2 crackers: 4.0 g

Sesame seeds, 2 tbsp.: 2.2 g

Wasa Fiber Crispbread, 2 crackers: 4.0 g

Wasa Lite Rye Crispbread, 2 crackers: 6.0 g

Whole Wheat Matzos, 1: 4.0 g

Grains and Pasta

Barley, 1/2 cup cooked: 3.0 g

Brown rice, 1/2 cup cooked: 2.0 g

Buckwheat, 1/2 cup cooked: 2.4 g

Bulgur, 1/2 cup cooked: 4.0 g

Macaroni, whole wheat, 1 cup cooked: 4.0 g

Oats, 1/2 cup cooked: 2.0 g

Oats, steel cut, 3 tbsp. dry: 3.0 g

Quinoa, 1/2 cup cooked: 2.6 g

Fruits

Apple with skin, 1 med.: 3.0 g

Apricots, 1/2 cup dried: 4.8 g

Banana, 1 med.: 3.0 g

Blackberries, 1 cup: 7.6 g

Blueberries, 1 cup: 3.5 g

Cantaloupe, 2 cups: 2.0 g

Cherries, 15: 2.0 g

Figs, 2 fresh: 3.0 g

Grapefruit, 1 whole: 3.2 g

Kiwi, 2 med.: 4.5 g

Orange, 1 med.: 3.0 g

Peach, 1 med.: 2.2 g

Pear, 1 med.: 5.5 g

Prunes, 5 dried: 3.4 g

Raspberries, 1 cup: 8.0 g

Strawberries, 1½ cups: 5.0 g

Vegetables

Acorn squash, ½ cup baked: 4.5 g

Artichoke, 1 med.: 7.0 g

Avocado, ¼ cup: 2.5 g

Broccoli, ½ cup cooked: 2.6 g

Broccoli, 1 cup chopped raw: 2.4 g

Brussels sprouts, 5: 3.8 g

Butternut squash, ½ cup baked: 3.3 g

Cabbage, 1 cup chopped raw: 2.2 g

Carrots, ½ cup cooked: 2.3 g

Carrots, 1 whole raw: 2.0 g

Collards, ½ cup cooked: 2.8 g

Corn, ½ cup cooked: 2.0 g

Green beans, 1 cup raw: 2.7 g

Green beans, ½ cup cooked: 2.0 g

Jicama, ½ cup raw: 3.2 g

Kale, 1 cup raw: 2.6 g

Lettuce, romaine, 2 cups: 2.0 g

Parsnips, ½ cup cooked: 2.8 g

Potato with skin, 1 sm. baked: 3.0 g

Spaghetti squash, 1 cup baked: 2.2 g

Sweet potato, 1 sm. baked: 2.0 g

Yam, ½ cup cooked: 2.6 g

Sample Menu Plans for Incorporating More Fiber in the Diet

The following outlines of sample menu plans offer one day of meals that will allow you to reach over 40 g of fiber in your diet. The items are eaten together as a meal or snack.

Sample Day A

Breakfast

½ cup Kasha Whole Grain Nuggets (7.0 g)

¼ cup nonfat milk, yogurt, or milk alternative

½ cup strawberries (1.7 g)

Snack

Hummus (3.7 g)

¼ cup raw jicama (1.6 g)

1 raw carrot (2.0 g)

Lunch

1 slice Ezekiel Sprouted Whole Grain Bread (3.0 g)

Turkey breast

1 cup Progresso Lentil Soup (5.0 g)

1 fresh apple with skin (3.0 g)

Snack

Organic nonfat or low-fat plain yogurt

1 tbsp. ground flaxseed (2.0 g)

½ cup blueberries (1.7 g)

½ cup raspberries (4.0 g)

Dinner

3 oz. baked salmon

½ cup baked acorn squash (4.5 g)

½ cup steamed broccoli (2.6 g)

Tossed green salad with vinaigrette dressing:

- 1 cup romaine lettuce (1.0 g)
- ½ cup raw cabbage (1.1 g)
- ¼ cup edamame (1.9 g)
- Cherry tomatoes (1.8 g)

2 fresh figs or 1 orange (3.0 g)

Total grams of fiber for this day: 44

Sample Day B

Breakfast

2 biscuits Shredded Wheat (6.0 g)

¼ cup nonfat milk, yogurt, or milk alternative

½ banana (1.5 g)

Snack

1 fresh peach (2.2 g)

Lunch

Large green salad with vinaigrette dressing:

- 2 cups romaine lettuce (2.0 g)
- ½ cup raw broccoli (1.2 g)
- ¼ cup kidney beans (3.3 g)

½ carrot (1.0 g)

½ cup raw cauliflower (1.0 g)

1 hardboiled egg (1.0 g)

Fresh fruit salad:

1 cup cantaloupe (1.0 g)

1½ cups strawberries (5.0 g)

Snack

2 Ryvita Sesame Rye crackers (4.0 g)

1 tbsp. almond butter

Dinner

Oven-roasted chicken breast

½ cup baked yam (2.6 g)

5 roasted brussels sprouts (3.8 g)

Fresh pear (5.5 g)

Total grams of fiber for this day: 44

Which Fish Have the Most EPA/DHA?

Fish are the ideal food to eat when trying to improve your diet. They are a rich source of high-quality protein, vitamins, minerals, and most importantly, the omega-3 fatty acids EPA and DHA. The benefits of eating fish are connected to their content of these important fatty acids. Since the 1980s, it has been well documented that consumption of fish is correlated with a lower risk of cardiovascular disease. More recently, research has demonstrated that regular fish consumption lowers the risk of certain cancers (breast, prostate, colon, and lung) and other chronic diseases such as diabetes, rheumatoid arthritis, and depression.

There are important safety issues to consider regarding fish consumption. The most common warning concerns mercury content, which is highest in certain tunas, swordfish, and shark. Mercury is toxic, and it accumulates in our bodies, which is particularly problematic for pregnant women and young children. FDA recommendations suggest that pregnant women or those who may become pregnant eat fresh tuna, swordfish, or shark no more than once per month. Fish considered safe for pregnant women include wild Pacific salmon, flounder, haddock, and farm-raised catfish and trout. Freshwater fish in general should be limited, as they are more likely to be contaminated with pesticides and potential carcinogens. Small deep-water fish are the best choice, with Alaskan salmon playing a starring role for both safety and omega-3 content.

Fish flesh contains variable amounts of the protective omega-3 fatty acids EPA and DHA. Fish that contain the highest amount of omega-3 fatty acids include salmon, bluefin tuna, herring, mackerel, and whitefish. Some fish that are high in omega-3 fatty acids, such as certain types of tuna, are not always the best choice due to their mercury content.

The best choices are those that are abundant, not endangered, and are caught or farmed in environmentally friendly ways. Common choices in this category include wild Alaskan salmon, Pacific cod, black cod, sardines, halibut, rainbow trout, tilapia, catfish, albacore and skipjack tuna, and striped bass, either farmed or wild.

The list below will give you some idea of which common fish or seafoods are the richest sources of EPA and DHA. To research a detailed list of fish and their safety levels of toxins, you can go to the websites www.montereybayaquarium.org and ewg.org.

The best and safest choices are in **bold**.

FISH	mg EPA+DHA per 100 g in 3½ oz., cooked
Anchovy	2055
Herring, Atlantic and Pacific	2014–2125
Pacific mackerel	1848
Salmon, sockeye, smoked, canned	**1570**
Tuna, bluefin	1477
Salmon, wild coho	**1374**
Salmon, canned, red, Alaskan	**1080**
Sardines	**984**
Rainbow trout	**988**
Striped bass	**967**
Flounder	**500**
Halibut	**463**
Tuna, canned light (safer than white)	**270**
Tuna, skipjack	**228**
Pacific cod	**215**

The Basic Plan for an Anti-inflammatory Diet

The purpose of this food plan is to help you achieve and maintain health by decreasing foods that lead to inflammation and pain, decreasing your intake of harmful chemicals, and optimizing your intake of healthy protein, fat, and carbs. It can also aid in weight management and in the prevention of heart attacks, type 2 diabetes, cancer, and strokes. The plan may be modified if you have food allergies or are gluten sensitive.

Grocery Shopping

Healthy food is really better for your body; it is not just a fad. It is best to do most of your food shopping at a market that offers a lot of organic and natural food choices. Buy organic fruits, vegetables, and milk products; eggs from free-range chickens; and grass-fed, grass-finished beef and lamb whenever possible. Non-organic fruits, vegetables, dairy, and meats contain pesticides and may contain other chemicals or harmful metals. These chemicals can be stored in your body, where they stimulate pain receptors, create inflammation, increase free radical production, and make it more difficult to heal.

Proteins

Your goal is to get sufficient healthy sources of protein to supply the amino acids that help preserve and build muscle and heal musculoskeletal tissues.

Protein is made from amino acids. Adequate protein is needed every day. It helps to maintain your muscles, and amino acids are a building block for many important cell reactions. Everyone needs at least 0.8 g of protein per kg of body weight (weight in pounds divided by 2.2).

Protein requirements

- For sedentary individuals: 0.8 g/kg of body weight
- When doing aerobic training that is moderate to vigorous: 1.2 g/kg of lean body weight
- When weight lifting to make body shaping or hypertrophy gains: 1.4–1.6 g/kg
- While healing from surgery: 1.0–1.2 g/kg
- For healing a tendon or ligament from an injury: 1.2 g/kg of lean weight

  Based on this scale, your protein needs are ________________.

Protein guidelines

- Have protein with each meal and snack if possible.
- Limit red meat or eliminate it unless it is free-range, grass-fed beef or lamb.
- Avoid charring or browning proteins and meats.
- Use organic meats or free-range meats and poultry (chicken and turkey) when possible.
- Use eggs from free-range chickens for protein.
- Avoid luncheon meats that have sodium nitrate or nitrites. Nitrate-free turkey is a good protein source.
- Use walnuts as a protein source for snacks and for their omega-3 fats.
- Use mixed nuts and seeds (pumpkin, sunflower).
- Consider adding nut butters (almond, cashew, macadamia) to breakfast cereal, bread, crackers, apples, and celery.
- Soy products, such as tempeh, miso, and soy milk, are good sources of protein if kept to one serving a day.
- If you are going to use milk products (milk, cheese, and yogurt), try to use organic milk products.
- For milk substitutes, you can use soy, rice, almond, or oat milk.
- Consider beans and grains (soy, millet, quinoa, lentils and other beans) as sources of protein and fiber.
- Get at least a third to a quarter of your daily protein need at breakfast by using a protein powder with whey or rice protein to make protein smoothies. You can blend 2 scoops in 10–12 oz. of a liquid with some organic berries (with or without a banana).
- Minimize eating large fish such as tuna and swordfish because of their mercury content. Avoid farm-raised salmon because of the PCB content; river trout is usually okay.

Fats

The goal is to eat healthy fats and decrease unhealthy fats. Your fat intake is directly related to inflammation. Follow these guidelines:

- Use coconut oil, canola oil, or olive oil (extra virgin is best) for cooking.
- Make your own salad dressing: 2 parts flaxseed oil, 4 parts extra virgin olive oil, and one part red wine vinegar or balsamic vinegar. You can add a small amount of toasted sesame for flavor.
- Use sources of omega-3 fats, including fresh ground flaxseeds and flaxseed oil (don't heat flaxseeds), sardines, wild salmon, and walnuts.
- Use a daily supplement of 1–4 g of high EPA/DHA fish oils (capsule or liquid), purified to eliminate mercury, pesticides, and so on.
- Use dry-roasted or raw nuts.
- Eliminate deep fried and breaded fried foods (french fries, Chicken McNuggets, etc.).
- Avoid all partially hydrogenated oils and trans fats by reading labels ("partially hydrogenated ___________oil").
- Decrease saturated fats (e.g., ice cream). Try to limit processed foods that have more than 6–8 g of fat per serving. Choose low-fat ice creams, low- or nonfat yogurt, and low- or healthy-fat salad dressings (vinaigrette, oil and vinegar).
- Choose leaner meats.
- Avoid highly heated fats, such as crispy bacon and french fries cooked in vats of oil.

Carbohydrates

The goal is to limit non-nutritive carbs and use healthy complex carbs as an energy and vitamin source.

- Have a daily intake of healthy and colorful fruits (berries, pomegranate, apples, pears, and citrus fruits) for fiber and beneficial phytochemicals to help your body quench free radicals and remove and detoxify toxins.
- Eat healthy vegetables daily (organic when possible), including cruciferous vegetables (broccoli, cabbage, cauliflower, kale), as they help your body detoxify.
- Eat other vegetables for their nutrients and fiber: chard, spinach, celery, squash, zucchini, cucumber.
- Eat from the onion family daily (onions, leeks, chard, garlic, chives), as these vegetables are good for connective tissue and detoxification.
- Consider juicing organic vegetables to improve your intake of phytochemicals: celery, apple, carrot, kale, broccoli, spinach, beets. Add some lemon or lime and some protein powder.
- Limit cookies, cakes, scones, muffins, potatoes, starches, sugars, rice, pasta, and breads unless you are training for a long aerobic event or do not have a weight management problem; in that case, use whole and sprouted grains in bread or boiled.
- Eat beans (kidney, black, pinto, garbanzo) for soluble fiber and to limit colon inflammation.
- Use a bread that has at least 3–5 g of protein and fiber per slice. Look for sprouted grain and seed breads. Use whole grain sources for carbs, such as quinoa and millet.
- Use a breakfast cereal that has at least 8 g of fiber and 4–10 g of protein per cup.

Food Additives

Try to avoid artificial colorings and diet beverages with aspartame. Minimize and avoid foods containing ingredients that have MSG or hidden MSG. To get a current list of hidden MSG in foods, do an online search for "MSG, hidden."

Steps for Healthier Food Choices

Start where you are and proceed step by step toward the goal. Follow these overall guidelines:

- Minimize or (ideally) eliminate partially hydrogenated oils in processed foods (use foods labeled "No Trans Fats").
- Minimize or avoid eating at fast food restaurants. At restaurants, choose butter-based toppings on the side, and eliminate sour cream and cream-based dishes. Choose salads (with oil and vinegar or vinaigrette) and vegetables, and avoid deep-fried entrées.
- Minimize or avoid deep-fried and breaded foods.
- Minimize sugars and starches (crackers, potatoes, rice, scones, cookies).
- Increase healthy fruits, such as apples and berries (have 2–3 servings per day).
- Use healthy veggies, such as those in the veggie list above (under "Carbohydrates"). Have a minimum of 3 servings per day.
- Try to choose organic fruits and veggies when your budget and the availability of these items allows.
- Eat protein at every meal.
- Purchase free-range poultry and meat (if you are not vegetarian).
- If you eat dairy products, choose low-fat, organic dairy products (milk, cheese, yogurt, ice cream).
- Use a good multivitamin and mineral supplement (taken at meals) that requires at least 2 per day, with minerals (calcium 500 mg per day and magnesium 500 mg per day) and antioxidants (A, C, E, selenium).
- Try some green tea daily.
- Minimize drinks with fructose and corn syrup.

- Choose veggie juices such as V8, or an organic version (Knudsen Very Veggie Organic, Lakeview Super Veggie).
- For fruit juice, choose one with a lot of phytonutrients and antioxidant-quenching abilities.
- If you are trying to lose weight, limit juices other than veggie juices to 4–6 oz. per day.

Breakfast Ideas

- Get at least a quarter of your daily protein needs met at breakfast.
- Make a protein smoothie (see “Protein” section above). Use enough protein powder to get 20–25 g.
- Use breakfast cereals that are high in protein and fiber, such as Nature’s Path Optimum Slim or Kashi Good Friends. Consider adding mixed nuts and fruit (blueberries, banana) to cereal.
- A 2- or 3-egg omelet or egg scramble with veggies (such as spinach, leeks, broccoli, tomatoes, or chives) is a good breakfast choice.

Breakfast

Nut butter oatmeal: Place 1 cup water, ⅓ cup steel-cut or old-fashioned oats and 2–3 chopped dates or 2 tbsp. raisins in a small saucepan. Bring to a boil. Reduce heat and simmer, stirring occasionally, for about 5 minutes. Add 1–2 tbsp. peanut or almond butter and mix well. Serve with 1 grated apple and a dollop of plain yogurt if desired.

Apple oatmeal: Place 1 cup steel-cut or old-fashioned rolled oats, 2 cups water, 2 small apples, washed and cut into bite-sized pieces, ¼ cup raisins or no-sugar-added dried berries, and 1 tsp. cinnamon together in a saucepan. Cover and cook over low heat for 20 minutes, stirring occasionally. This makes 2–3 servings.

Homemade granola: Mix together the following: 1 lb. rolled oats, 2 cups oat bran, 1 cup grated coconut, 1 cup chopped pecans, ¼ cup sesame seeds, ½ cup sunflower seeds, ⅓ cup oil, ½ cup agave nectar or stevia to taste. Spread a thin layer about ½ in. thick on an unoiled cookie sheet and bake at 350°F for 20 minutes or until golden brown. Stir occasionally during the baking to assure even browning. Remove from oven and add unsweetened dried fruit if desired; mix well. Let cool before storing. (This makes many servings; limit portion to ½ cup per meal. Serve dry or with almond or rice milk.)

Berry smoothie: Blend in a blender: 1 cup rice or almond milk, 1–2 scoops powdered protein of choice (to equal 15–25 g protein), ½ cup ice cubes if using fresh fruit, ½ cup strawberries, ½ cup blueberries, 1–2 tbsp. ground flaxseed, 1–2 tbsp. nut butter (optional).

Super smoothie: 1 cup diluted cranberry juice (half water, half juice), ¼ cup fresh or frozen cranberries, ¾ cup frozen blueberries, 1 scoop whey protein, 1 tbsp. flaxseed oil, 1 tbsp. ground flaxseed, stevia to taste if desired. Combine all ingredients in the blender. Mix until smooth and creamy, or for about 1–2 minutes. (Change to strawberries and raspberries instead of blueberries for variety, and/or add ½ cup plain yogurt instead of whey protein if desired.)

Oat crepes: Place ⅓ cup rolled oats, ⅓ cup almond or rice milk, and 1 egg in the blender and blend until smooth. The batter will be thin. Drop the batter by the ¼ cup or less onto a hot, lightly oiled skillet or crepe pan. Cook over medium-high heat until set and golden brown on the bottom. Turn and cook briefly on the other side. Top with fresh berries and plain yogurt and 2 tbsp. pecans, walnuts, or almonds.

Lunch Ideas

- Have a sandwich with high-fiber, high-protein sprouted grain bread (see "Carbohydrates" section above). In your sandwich, have nut butter (such as almond, macadamia, or cashew), turkey or chicken (with no nitrates), or organic cheese, along with veggies (lettuce, tomatoes, olives, cucumber, onions).
- If you have a salad for lunch, add healthy protein, such as beans (kidney, garbanzo, pinto), sliced nitrate-free turkey, wild salmon, or organic cottage cheese. Use numerous colorful veggies in your salad and try to include cruciferous veggies such as broccoli. Use an oil and vinegar salad dressing or make your own (see "Fats" above).

Dinner Ideas

- Try to have 2 servings of healthy veggies and a lowfat protein source.
- Minimize desserts (other than fruit).

Lunch and Dinner

Spinach and garlic salad: Place 1 or 2 garlic cloves into an ovenproof dish and add 2 tbsp. olive oil. Roast in a 375°F oven for 15–20 minutes. Transfer the garlic and olive oil into a salad bowl. Add 1 lb. organic spinach, ½ cup chopped walnuts, and 2 tsp. lemon juice, and toss well to coat the salad. Season with salt and pepper to taste.

Stir-fried greens: Cut up 8 scallions, 2 celery stalks, 1 cup white radishes, and 1½ cup sugar snap peas or snow peas into strips. Shred 1½ cups napa cabbage and ½ cup bok choy or spinach. Heat 1 tbsp. olive oil and 1 tbsp. sesame oil together in a wok and add the garlic. Add the other cut vegetables to the wok and stir-fry for about 2 minutes. Then add the cabbage and bok choy or spinach to the skillet and stir-fry for another minute or so. Add 1 tsp. finely grated fresh gingerroot and pepper to taste, and cook another minute. This is great with kale and other miscellaneous greens of your choosing.

Rice and beans: Cook 1 cup brown or wild rice according to the package directions and set aside. Heat 2 tbsp. olive oil in a skillet and add green and red peppers, one each, chopped, and one chopped onion. Cook for 5 minutes or until soft. Add 1 small red or green chili, chopped, and 2 chopped tomatoes, and cook for another 2–3 minutes. Add this vegetable mixture and 1 cup canned red kidney beans, rinsed and drained, to the rice and stir to mix. Add 1 tbsp. chopped fresh basil, 2 tsp. chopped fresh thyme, and 1 tsp. Cajun spice (such as Tony Chachere's) and mix well. Add sea salt and pepper to taste.

Black bean soup: In a 3-quart pot, heat 1 tbsp. olive oil over medium heat, add 1 medium chopped onion and 2 minced garlic cloves, and cook until tender. Stir in 2 tsp. chili powder, 1 tsp. ground cumin, 2 cans black beans, rinsed and drained, 1 can organic vegetable broth, and 1 cup water, and heat to boiling. Reduce heat to low and simmer for 15 minutes. Use a handheld mixer to blend the soup to a creamy consistency. Garnish with ½ cup chopped cilantro and lime wedges. Add avocado for garnish as well, if desired.

Hot lentil salad: Cook one cup brown or green lentils according to package instructions. Heat 4 tbsp. olive oil in a pan, and cook one small sliced onion with 4 stalks of sliced celery, 2 garlic cloves, crushed or grated, 2 diced zucchinis, and ¾ cup fresh green beans cut into small lengths. Cook for 5 minutes, then add ½ a red bell pepper and a yellow bell pepper, diced, to the pan and cook for another minute. Stir in 1 tsp. Dijon mustard and 1 tbsp. balsamic vinegar. Pour the warm mixture over the cooked lentils and toss together well. Season with salt and pepper to taste.

Chicken jambalaya: Cook 3 oz. brown rice as directed on package and set aside. Heat 1–2 tbsp. olive oil in a heavy skillet and cook 2 large (6–8 oz.) chicken breasts, diced, until brown, about 3 minutes on each side. Add another 1–2 tbsp. olive oil to the pan and cook 2 cloves crushed garlic and 1 small red onion, chopped, for about 2–3 minutes. Add 1 diced eggplant, 1 diced green bell pepper, ½ cup frozen peas, and 1 cup broccoli florets and cook for another 5 minutes. Stir in 1 cup organic vegetable broth, 8 oz. fresh or canned chopped tomatoes, 1 tbsp. tomato paste, 1 tsp. Creole seasoning, and ½ tsp. chili flakes. Add salt and pepper to taste and cook for 15–20 minutes. Stir in the rice and chicken and cook until hot.

Stuffed peppers: Halve 4 green peppers and place in an oven-safe dish. Mix together 2 cups cooked long grain brown or wild rice, 1 can organic stewed tomatoes, one small onion, chopped, 1 cup chopped fresh mushrooms, 2 tbsp. fresh basil, and salt and pepper to taste. Stuff the pepper halves with the rice mixture so that each pepper contains an even amount. Bake in the oven at 350°F for 30 minutes or until peppers are tender.

Vegetable soup: In a large saucepan sprayed with nonstick cooking spray, sauté 1 cup sliced carrots, 1 cup diced onion, and 2–4 minced garlic cloves over low heat until soft, about 5 minutes. Add 4 cups (32 oz.) organic broth (beef, chicken, or vegetable), 2–3 cups diced green cabbage, 1 cup green beans, ½ can no-salt-added tomato paste, ½ tbsp. dried basil, ¼ tbsp. oregano, and ¼ tbsp. salt. Bring to a boil. Lower heat and simmer, covered, about 15 minutes or until beans are tender. Stir in ½ cup diced zucchini and heat 3–4 minutes. Serve hot. Add other vegetables and legumes as desired.

Portobello steaks: You'll need 6 portobello mushroom caps, ½ cup fresh squeezed lemon juice, 2 tbsp. apple cider vinegar, 2 tbsp. pure maple syrup, 2 tsp. fresh grated ginger, and ½ tsp. marjoram. Wash mushrooms and place in a gallon-size plastic sealable bag. Combine remaining ingredients in a bowl and stir to combine. Add to the mushrooms and marinate for a few hours. Grill indoors or out until cooked through. Serve with baked sweet potatoes and grilled squash and asparagus.

Grilled vegetables: Toss yellow squash, zucchini, and asparagus with 2 tbsp. extra virgin olive oil. Salt and pepper to taste. Grill indoors or out until tender.

Roasted vegetables: Take a variety of raw non-starchy vegetables, washed and prepared in medium-sized portions. Place in a 9 × 13 in. roasting pan. Drizzle with olive oil, add minced garlic, and salt and pepper to taste. Roast at 375–400°F for 20–30 minutes, stirring every 15 minutes until desired tenderness.

Baked sweet potatoes: Wash sweet potatoes, prick with a fork several times, and place in a 400°F oven for an hour. Less time may be needed if potatoes are small.

Vegetarian spaghetti squash: Slice squash in half lengthwise. Scoop out the seeds with a spoon as you would a pumpkin. Then completely submerge both halves in boiling water and cook for about 20–25 minutes, or until the inside is tender to a fork and pulls apart in strands. (It is better to undercook if you are not sure.) Remove, drain, and cool with cold water or an ice bath to stop the cooking. Then use a fork to scrape the cooked squash out of its skin, and at the same time, fluff and separate the squash into spaghetti-like strands. Discard the skin. Reheat the squash strands by dipping with a strainer in boiling water just before serving.

You can also bake the spaghetti squash in the oven. Just scoop seeds out as described above and prick outside skin with a fork. Place skin-side-up in a baking pan with 1 in. water. Bake 45 minutes or until tender in a 400°F oven. Remove and allow to cool for a few minutes until they can be handled. Scrape with a fork as mentioned above and serve with stir-fry sauce.

Stir-fry sauce: You will need 10 Roma tomatoes, peeled, seeded, and chopped coarsely (or you may use two 14-oz. cans of petite diced or crushed tomatoes, unsalted if possible), 2 cups thinly sliced mushrooms, 2 cloves garlic, 2 cups chopped broccoli florets or 1 package baby spinach, 2 tsp. oregano (powdered or flakes), and sea salt to taste. Sauté mushrooms and onion with garlic and oregano. Add tomatoes and other vegetables. Cook until tender and heated through. Toss in a large bowl with spaghetti squash strands. Serve hot. Makes about 6 servings.

Snacks

Hummus: In a food processor, combine two 15-oz. cans garbanzo beans, drained and rinsed, 4 cloves mashed garlic, ⅔ cup tahini, ½ cup water, ¼ cup olive oil, and the juice of a large lemon. Blend until smooth. Add salt, starting at ½ tsp. and adding to taste. Place this hummus mixture into a serving dish and sprinkle with toasted pine nuts and chopped parsley. This can be served with carrots, celery, cucumbers, jicama, bell peppers, or any other vegetables, as well as with blue corn chips or any type of healthy crackers.

Guacamole: Cut two avocados in half and remove the pits. Scoop out flesh with a spoon and place in a food processor. Add ½ cup fresh cilantro, 1 clove garlic, and juice of half a lemon, and puree in the food processor. Add 4–5 chopped cherry tomatoes and season with sea salt to taste.

Homemade pickles: Chop 1 large cucumber into slices, add half a small sliced yellow onion, and mix with 3–4 tbsp. fresh dill. Mix 1 cup apple cider vinegar and 1 cup water in a container with a tight lid. Add the vegetables. Let the cucumber and onion marinate for at least 4 hours in the refrigerator before eating. This will keep in the refrigerator for at least one week. Add sea salt and pepper to taste.

Cinnamon apples: Core 1 medium red apple into slices and place in a microwave-safe dish. Pour 1 tsp. cinnamon mixed with 1 tbsp. water over the chopped apples and microwave for 45–60 seconds. Add one packet of stevia to the warmed apple if desired.

Balsamic vinegar and fruit: Pit and quarter 3–4 of your favorite stone fruits, such as peaches, plums, or nectarines, and place in an oven-safe dish. Drizzle balsamic vinegar over the fruit and bake at 400°F for 15–20 minutes. Remove fruit and garnish with fresh mint leaves.

Roasted nuts: Take 2 cups of your favorite nuts, preferably walnuts or pecans, and lightly coat with 1 tbsp. olive oil. Spread nuts on a baking sheet and place in the oven for 10–12 minutes at 350°F. Stir nuts halfway through baking for even browning. Watch nuts carefully—they burn easily. Let nuts cool and add a small amount of sea salt to taste if desired. They are great even without salt.

Cookbooks and Food Books with Recipes: A Reading List

Allergy and Candida Cooking: Understanding and Implementing Plans for Healing, 3rd edition, Sondra K. Lewis with Dorie Fink (Canary Connect, 2005)

Chakra Foods for Optimum Health, Deanna Minich (Conari Press, 2009)

Cooking Vegetarian, Joseph Forest and Vesanto Mellina, RD (Macmillan, 1996)

Eat, Drink, and Weigh Less, Mollie Katzen and Walter Willet, MD (Hyperion, 2006)

Farmer John's Cookbook: The Real Dirt on Vegetables, Farmer John Peterson and Angelic Organics (Gibbs Smith, 2006)

Feeding the Whole Family: Cooking with Whole Food, 3rd edition, Cynthia Lair, with foreword by Peggy O'Mara (Sasquatch Books, 2008)

Flying Apron's Gluten-Free & Vegan Baking Book, Jennifer Katzinger (Sasquatch Books, 2009)

The Gluten-Free Almond Flour Cookbook, Elana Amsterdam (Celestial Arts, 2009)

Gluten-Free, Sugar-Free Cooking, Susan O'Brien (Marlowe and Co., 2006)

The Gluten-Free Vegan, Susan O'Brien (Da Capo Press, 2007)

Healing with Whole Foods, Paul Pitchford (North Atlantic Books, 1993)

The New Becoming Vegetarian: The Essential Guide to a Healthy Vegetarian Diet, Vesanto Melina, MS, RD, and Brenda Davis, RD (Healthy Living Publications, 2003)

The New Moosewood Cookbook. Mollie Katzen (Ten Speed Press, 2000)

Simple Treats: A Wheat-Free Dairy-Free Guide to Scrumptious Baked Goods. Ellen Abraham (Book Publishing Co., 2003)

The UltraMetabolism Cookbook: 200 Delicious Recipes That Will Turn on Your Fat-Burning DNA. Mark Hyman, MD (Scribner, 2007)

The UltraSimple Diet: Kick-Start Your Metabolism and Safely Lose up to 10 lbs in 7 Days. Mark Hyman, MD (Pocket Books, 2007)

Vegetarian Cooking for People with Allergies, Raphael Rettner, DC (Book Publishing Co., 1997)

Vegetarian Family Cookbook, Nava Atlas (Broadway Books, 2004)

The Whole Life Nutrition Cookbook: Whole Foods Recipes for Personal and Planetary Health, 2nd edition, Alissa Segersten and Tom Malterre, MS, CN (Whole Life Press, 2007)

YOU on a Diet: The Owner's Manual for Waist Management, Michael F. Roizen, MD, and Mehmet C. Oz, MD (Free Press, 2006)

Detoxification

Suggestions for Decreasing Toxicity and Harmful Chemical Exposures

Certain chemicals applied to your skin or in the air can be absorbed by your body and may cause harm to your cells and organ systems. They can cause inflammation and increase the body's production of free radicals, thus increasing your likelihood of developing chronic health problems. The following information will help you decrease your exposure to toxicity.

Food

- Shift your food purchases and consumption to organic when possible. It is most important to use organic dairy products (milk, cheese, yogurt, ice cream, etc.). Free-range meats and eggs are desirable to purchase as organic. Minimize the use of large fish (swordfish, tuna, etc.), as they are higher in mercury.

- Purchase organic strawberries and apples, and refer to the Environmental Working Group (www.ewg.org/foodnews/) or Consumer Reports websites to stay current about which fruits and veggies are most important to eat organic.

Hair

- For hair products (including shampoo and colors), look for products without alcohol, sodium lauryl sulfate, parabens, phthalates, and other petrochemicals. Check your local yellow pages and magazines to see if there is an environmentally oriented hair salon in your area.
- Avoid using hairspray.
- Avoid perfumes or other skin or hair care products that use synthetic fragrances.

Skin Care and Makeup

- Use low-toxin makeup and skin creams (avoid products with phthalates, parabens, propylene glycol, alcohols, and fragrances). In general, skin care products from health food stores without the above ingredients are a safer bet.
- Consider using antioxidant creams on your skin: low-solvent products with CoQ10, vitamin C, and botanical squalene.

Antiperspirants and Deodorants

Avoid aluminum-containing antiperspirants and antacids. Since virtually all antiperspirants contain aluminum, it may be advisable to minimize or discontinue use.

Water

Water can harbor many toxins.

- Regular consumption of unfiltered water can significantly contribute to the toxic load of your body.
- Water quality will vary from city to city, but in general it is better to filter tap water with a multi-stage carbon filter or reverse osmosis filter.
- Try to avoid bottled water in soft plastic containers, as the plastics often leach into the water. Minimize the use of plastic water bottles that have been in a hot car.
- Minimize the use of CamelBak-type plastic hydration backpacks.
- Mineral waters in glass bottles are generally safe, unless there is a question of the quality of the source.
- Drink approximately 6–8 glasses of water or healthy liquids each day. Use glass or ceramic when possible.
- Filter shower water in order to limit your exposure to chlorinated hydrocarbons.

Plastics

Plastics can disrupt hormones in your body.

- Avoid plastic bottles and containers with the numbers 3, 6, and 7 on the bottom. These are most likely to leach plastics into the food, juice, or water that they contain.
- Buy juices and water in glass containers when possible.
- Avoid soft vinyl plastic (PVCs), such as plastic shower curtains, hydration packs, vinyl raincoats, and toys.
- Do not microwave food in plastic containers.
- Minimize washing plastic containers in the dishwasher under high heat.
- Minimize the use of cling wrap; try to use paper or cloth wraps.

Dental Care

Pick a dentist who is aware of healthy choices for the mouth—perhaps a more holistic or biologically oriented dentist who does not fill cavities with new mercury fillings.

- Avoid mercury amalgam fillings.
- Get a second opinions on root canals.
- Avoid if possible having two different metals in adjacent teeth.

Home and Cleaning Products

Make your home a source of health.

- Purchase the most natural cleaning and other household products you can find. Avoid spraying pesticides or herbicides in your home and on your property.
- Use only green and low-volatile organic compounds (VOC) products in a remodel or a new home.
- Avoid furniture made of particle board, or buy used furniture that has had a chance to off-gas.
- Let a new car off-gas by keeping the windows open.
- Use an air filter such as a high-efficiency particulate air (HEPA) filter with a charcoal filter to clean the debris in the air.
- Minimize the amount of regular carpet in your home, or use natural carpets.
- Avoid using pesticides in your house.
- When remodeling your home or office, use a low- or no-VOC paint, carpet or rug.
- Minimize carpet and choose hardwoods, but not laminates (avoid Pergo, for example).
- Take off shoes at the door to decrease indoor chemicals and pesticides.

- Avoid urea formaldehyde in building products.
- Change the filter on your furnace every three months, using the best allergy furnace filter you can find.

Electromagnetic Fields

People with headaches, neck pain, or shoulder pain should decrease their exposure to low-level electromagnetic fields.

- Minimize your cell phone use.
- Minimize your use of portable phones at home and shift to corded phones.
- Take the clock radio away from the head of your bed.
- Get the electromagnetic fields measured in a potential new car before you buy it.

Website References

These are my favorite websites to help educate you on environmental chemicals.

Environmental Working Group, www.ewg.org

Toxic-Free Future, www.watoxics.org

Plastics for kitchen use: www.greenguide.co.uk

Database of links and information about plastics and other environmental issues: mindfulofthehome.com/use-less-plastic/

Lifestyle Changes for Adrenal Stress Syndrome

Lifestyle changes to help if you have been under prolonged stress:

Avoiding Adrenal Stimulators

It is very important to avoid certain foods and chemicals in order to avoid excessive stress on the adrenal glands. In order to normalize the adrenals, not only is nutritional support required, but the removal of stimulants and sources of adrenal stress need to be eliminated as well. People who do not comply by avoiding stimulators will have minimal results. The following is a list of foods and chemicals that need to be completely avoided when making an attempt to normalize adrenal function.

- Concentrated sugars
- Caffeine
- Nicotine
- Alcohol
- Allergenic foods (histamine is an adrenal stimulant)
- Partially hydrogenated fats (they inhibit steroid hormone synthesis)
- Artificial sweeteners (they block the conversion of phenylalanine to tyrosine, which is needed to synthesize catecholamines in the adrenal medulla)
- Overtraining
- Inadequate sleep

Stabilize Glucose Levels

If blood glucose levels are not stabilized, there will be minimal results when attempting to correct adrenal status. This is especially a concern with people who have reactive hypoglycemia symptoms, such as irritability before meals, getting "shaky" and lightheaded when meals are missed, and relief of fatigue after eating. When blood sugar levels fall, healthy adrenals restore the levels back to normal. If the stress to the adrenal glands is not removed, the adrenals will not have the opportunity to rebuild. In addition to supplying the adrenals with the nutrients they require to stabilize blood glucose levels, dietary guidelines need to be addressed to stabilize blood sugar levels throughout the day.

- Do not skip breakfast. If your adrenals are healthy and strong and you do not suffer from fatigue, then the intermittent fasting diet may work really well for you.
- Eat a high-quality, protein-based breakfast.
- Eat every 2–3 hours. Do not wait until you are hungry.
- Snack with low glycemic foods, such as nuts, seeds, and hard-boiled eggs.
- Drink fruit juices, carrot juice, and V8 juice in small amounts, 6 oz. or less.
- Never consume high glycemic foods (e.g., fruit) without consuming a source of protein at the same time.
- Avoid all adrenal stimulants (as listed above).
- Eat a well-balanced diet consisting mostly of vegetables, quality grains, and lean meats.

Exercise in Aerobic Heart Range

We have two systems of energy production in our bodies—aerobic and anaerobic. *Anaerobic exercise* includes activities that require fast explosive movements, such as weightlifting, fast-paced jogging, sprinting, and any other form of exercise that cannot be performed for a long duration. Anaerobic activity will put excess stress on the adrenals because simple sugars are being used for energy. When sugar levels decrease, the adrenals are required to normalize blood sugar levels.

On the other hand, *aerobic exercise* includes long-duration activities such as walking, slow jogging, slow cycling, and any other form of exercise that involves endurance. It is crucial for patients with either hyperadrenia (increased cortisol) or hypoadrenia (low cortisol) to exercise in the aerobic heart range. Aerobic exercise utilizes the fat-burning system of the body instead of the sugar-burning system induced by anaerobic activity. Aerobic activity will not only decrease cortisol levels but will also use fatty acids for energy instead of simple sugars and will not require the stress put on the adrenal glands to normalize blood sugar levels during and after the workout.

Relaxation Techniques

Simple and quick relaxation and mental imaging techniques can be very helpful in reducing the mental effects of stress on people with adrenal stress syndrome. The stressful occurrences of daily life can have an adverse impact on the adrenal glands. Although each person has different levels of stress and a different reaction to stress, the mental aspect of relaxation cannot be overlooked. This is especially important with those of us who have a high load of emotional or mental stress. Here are a couple of techniques that may be beneficial in such situations. I recommend these exercises to all my patients who require relaxation from stress. Each exercise must be carried out in a quiet and restful atmosphere.

Exercise 1: Positive Mental Imaging

Think about the stressful events of the day. Try to put yourself back in the moment while utilizing as many senses as possible. Once one of the stressful events has been established, recreate the scenario while adding humorous and cartoon-like features to the people in the scene. For example, if you had a negative experience of being scolded by your boss, picture your boss with a big nose and goofy ears until the scenario becomes humorous. Go through all the stressful images from your day, incorporating positive imagery into each one of the scenes.

Exercise 2: Muscle Contraction and Relaxation

Lie on your back with your eyes closed. Contract a group of muscles maximally for two seconds. Start with the facial muscles and go up and down the body with different muscle groups, such as the quadriceps, hamstrings, calf muscles, toes, abdominals, pectorals, biceps, triceps, forearms, fingers, and so on. Continue until you have gone through each muscle group two or three times. When finished with this exercise, continue to lie on your back and take deep long breaths as long as desired.

Suggestions for Better Sleep

Minimize or Avoid Stimulants

Many substances or routines that we participate in on a daily basis can interfere with our sleep. The simplest place to start when wanting to improve your sleep is to avoid certain stimulants.

- Avoid alcohol (wine, beer, and hard liquor) within three hours of bedtime.
- Avoid caffeine-containing beverages or foods after 2:00 p.m. If you are sensitive to caffeine, avoid it after noon. These items include Pepsi, Coke, Mountain Dew, tea, coffee, lattes, chocolate, and coffee- or espresso-containing ice creams and desserts. Read the labels of everything you eat and drink!
- Avoid Sudafed or other decongestant cold medicines at night.
- Some medications may have stimulating effects. Consult your pharmacist and doctor to determine whether any of them might be contributing to sleep problems. Do not discontinue them without permission from your doctor.
- Complete any aerobic exercise before 6:00 p.m. (or at least three hours before bedtime).

Nighttime Tension and Anxiety

Avoid anxiety-provoking activities close to bedtime:

- Avoid watching the news before going to bed.
- Avoid reading stimulating, exciting materials in bed.

- Avoid paying bills before bed.
- Avoid checking your financial reports or the stock market before bedtime.
- Avoid arguments before bedtime.
- Schedule difficult conversations well before bedtime—preferably at least three hours before.
- Try to achieve some action plan or resolution of a discussion or argument before trying to go to sleep.

Sleep Planning and Bedroom Preparation

Plan your sleep by putting it into your schedule; plan for eight and a half to nine hours in bed.

- As much as possible, go to sleep and wake up at the same time each day. This will help train your biological clock.
- Go to bed before midnight, as late-hour sleep is not as helpful as earlier sleep.
- Avoid late afternoon or evening naps.
- Avoid naps longer than forty-five minutes, unless you are sick or quite sleep deprived.
- Avoid large meals or spicy foods before bed.
- Finish all eating three hours prior to going to sleep.
- Avoid drinking more than 4–8 oz. of fluid before going to bed.
- Take a hot salt or soda aromatherapy bath. Raising your body temperature before sleep helps induce sleep. A hot bath also relaxes muscles and reduces tension. Add 1–2 cups of a mixture of Epsom salts (magnesium sulfate absorbed through the skin is very relaxing) and ½ to 1 cup baking soda (sodium bicarbonate is alkalizing to a stressed-out acidic body) to 10 drops lavender oil (helps lower cortisol levels).

Trouble Falling Asleep or Staying Asleep

There are strategies to use if you have trouble falling asleep or staying asleep.

- Consider reading a good book under low light to help with falling asleep.
- Don't stay in bed more than 20–30 minutes trying to fall asleep. Leave your bedroom and go to a relaxing room other than the bedroom and read or do a relaxation technique such as meditation.
- If you awaken early because of light, put a dark covering over your eyes.
- If you awaken early because of recurrent thoughts, try writing them in a journal. If this does not help, consider counseling. Depression might be a factor.

Bedroom Air Quality

Consider the quality of the air you are breathing at night.

- Keep your bedroom air clean, especially if you have nasal congestion or are prone to snoring. Use HEPA or other types of air purifiers or filters to clean the air in your bedroom. Use the filter on a low setting at night if the noise is soothing. Otherwise use the filter on a medium setting for 4–6 hours during the day.
- Consider cleaning the vents in your house once a year; change your furnace filters every three months.
- Avoid toxic glues or other items producing an odor.
- If you see mold or smell mustiness in your bedroom, have it cultured for mold with culture plates. If there is mold, have the house evaluated for water leaks and air quality issues that need to be fixed and see that the mold is cleaned appropriately.

- If your nose is blocked, giving you trouble breathing, take the above steps and consider using a saline spray before bed. Also consider some type of breathe-easy strips on your nose. Make sure you read the instructions and fit the strips over the lower third of your nose.

Light, Noise, Temperature, and Environmental Issues

Other factors may be keeping you awake.

- Turn down the light in the bathroom and in rooms you are in fifteen minutes before going to bed.
- Decrease the light in your bedroom by using a dimmer or a reading light with a dimmer.
- Use dark window shades or a set of eye shades or a black covering for your eyes when trying to sleep or if you awaken too early because of light.
- Decrease irritating noises in your space by closing windows or using ear plugs, or using a white noise generator or a HEPA air filter.
- Turn off or remove any appliances or clocks that make a noise.
- Make sure your sleeping area is the correct temperature range (not too hot or too cold).
- Avoid sleeping near electric fields. Try to have your head at least five feet away from electric fields, if possible. Possible sources of electrical fields include electrical outlets, clock radios, stereos, computers, and monitors. Consider moving these devices or moving your bed or your position in the bed. Consider using a TriField EMF Meter or other meter to test for these fields.
- Avoid sleeping on a water bed or an electric mattress because of the excessive heat and the electric fields.

Ongoing Nighttime Tension and Anxiety

There are further strategies you can consider for dealing with ongoing anxiety about sleeping.

- Avoid repeated negative judgments about the fact that you are unable to sleep.
- Use positive self-talk phrases regarding your ability to relax and fall asleep: "I can fall asleep." "I can relax." "Any amount of sleep I get is just fine."
- Try writing in your journal any disturbing thoughts that are running through your mind.
- Schedule a time within the next few days to deal with whatever is troubling you. If you are having trouble managing your concerns for more than a few weeks, consult your healthcare provider for treatment suggestions or a counseling or therapy referral.
- Many relaxing yoga or stress-reducing mindful breathing CDs and DVDs are available. Use one to help you find a relaxing bedtime ritual that works for you.

Bedding and Pillows

Your bedding could be part of the problem.

- Consider replacing your pillows with hypoallergenic pillows. Use ultrafine allergy pillow and mattress covers.
- Consider using a "side sleeper" pillow for under your neck when sleeping on your side.
- Consider using a body pillow to hug and put between your knees to align your back and shoulders at night.
- Roll backwards at a slight angle onto a body pillow if you have hip bursitis.
- Sleep on the highest quality bed linens you can afford.

Supplements and Light

Consider taking natural support at bedtime.

- Consider 1–5 mg of melatonin to fall asleep and/or 5–20 mg time-released melatonin to stay asleep.
- Take 50–300 mg of 5-HTP one hour before bedtime.
- Take 500–2000 mg of taurine one hour before bedtime.
- Take a magnesium-calcium supplement at bedtime; a ratio of 250 mg to 500 mg is a typical dose. Alternatively, take 400–800 mg of magnesium citrate or magnesium glycinate.
- Take calming herbs—lemon balm, passion flower, or valerian root, as a tea, supplement, or tincture.
- Establish an evening herbal tea habit to support relaxation and sleep onset.
- Consider half an hour of exposure to a blue or 10,000 lux bright light (first thing in the morning) if you are going to bed too late and want to shift to an earlier bedtime.

Resources to Help You with Healthy Eating

Organic Food

www.thrivemarket.com

www.sunorganicfarm.com

www.theorganicpages.com

Healthy Meal Delivery

Sun Basket, www.sunbasket.com

Peter's Paleo, www.petespaleo.com

Organic Herb Teas

www.mightyleaf.com

www.choiceorganicteas.com

www.yogitea.com

www.republicoftea.com

www.numitea.com

Water

Aquatru: Water filters-reverse osmosis, www.aquatruwater.com

www.brita.com

The Biome Medic Supplement to Clear Glyphosate

Biome Medic supplement is specifically formulated to heal the gut microbiome from the effects of glyphosate (Roundup). It both chelates and expels toxins and feeds the gut with vital minerals and prebiotics to support the regeneration of the microvilli and aerobic bacteria colonies.

This protocol floods the cells with high-potency superfood nutrition, restores the gut microbiome, and acts to detoxify glyphosate and toxins, and clear mold, fungus, yeast, and parasites. These combined functions allow the body to heal and rebalance the negative effects of toxic overload.

Biome Medic is best taken twice a day for at least six weeks, then regularly for maintenance after that. Start with one twice a day for ten days, then two twice a day for ten days for more intensive detoxification, and then continue with one twice a day. A four-pack is best and the best price. (To order, use these links: four-pack bit.ly/37MIOFZ; single bit.ly/38YlSDW, or contact Leiah Lauren Borowsky, L.Ac, LMT, CYT, www.EnliveningSpirit.com, 510-816-8027.)

PEMF/Physical Vascular Device and Electroceuticals

Linda Hetzel

Health & Wellness Navigator

Independent BEMER Distributor

415-328-5060

Linda@LindaHetzel.com

Sauna

Relax Sauna

Sunlight Sauna

Environmentally Clean Home

supernaturalmom.com

"Simple Ways to Protect Yourself from EMFs and 5G Cellular Wireless" (supernaturalmom.com/emfebook/)

JACQUELINE CHAN, DO, MIM

Jacqueline Chan, DO, MIM, is an osteopathic physician with more than 20 years of experience as a cutting-edge integrative holistic doctor. Dr. Chan acts as a synergist, combining the tenets of her osteopathic training to balance the structure of the body and prevent and optimize health through diet and lifestyle. She utilizes both functional medicine lab work (to identify factors that put her clients at risk of autoimmune or degenerative conditions) and energy medicine (to assist in balancing the energy centers of the body). She has recently enhanced her practice by developing an intuitive assessment of the body based on energy medicine.

Dr. Chan's main interest is in total-body rejuvenation for peak performance and longevity. She enjoys helping those who want to perform optimally in all areas of their lives and prevent degenerative or life-threatening illnesses such as cancer, Alzheimer's, or autoimmune conditions. Dr. Chan likes to address the physical organ systems, emotional health, psychic health, and structural health of the body through hands-on osteopathic assessment, kinesiology, energy medicine, and lab work. Dr. Chan believes in the basic tenet that complex chronic health issues can be healed if we think outside the box by identifying and eliminating stressors to the physiological system. Such stressors include toxin build-up, hormone imbalances, and stealth pathogens (viruses, fungus, mold, Lyme disease, and parasites). Simultaneous with clearing stressors out of the system is the optimization of a person's health by balancing the central nervous system. This is accomplished through an individualized approach to the immune system, gut and microbiome function, genetic frailties, diet, and lifestyle factors with the main tools of nutrition, a sophisticated application of nutraceuticals and herbal remedies, and osteopathic manual medicine.

Dr. Jacqueline Chan received her BA in philosophy with honors from Mount Holyoke College in Massachusetts. She worked on Wall Street in banking before deciding that was not her true calling. She then earned her doctorate of osteopathy from Ohio University College of Osteopathic Medicine in 1997, graduating in the top ten, and received her family-practice-emphasis internship and residency at Doctors Hospital in Columbus, Ohio, in 2000. She is board certified in integrative holistic medicine and neuromusculoskeletal medicine. She has appeared with Dr. Oz on Sheila Gale's radio show on and *Legendary Leaders* radio shows. In 2012 she collaborated on a research study on chronic disease with Beverly Rubik, PhD, at the Institute of Frontier Science in Berkeley, California.

In 2013 she graduated from the Academy of Intuition Medicine, where she is now on faculty. She also became an adjunct faculty member at the Energy Medicine University in 2017.

Dr. Chan's goal is to connect her patients with their truth, their wisdom, and their own innate healing force. As a holistic medicine physician, she believes that compassion, presence, and grace are crucial healing forces, along with intelligently applied clinical knowledge. Her hobbies include hiking, meditating, dancing, writing poetry, horseback riding, and traveling.

To contact Dr. Chan or to schedule an appointment, please visit her website at www.drjacqueline.com.

DR. JACQUELINE CHAN'S SERVICES

I describe all my client services on my website, www.drjacqueline.com. Please contact me at drjacqueline.com.

ACKNOWLEDGMENTS

I am greatly indebted to the inspirational teachings of cranial osteopathy, functional medicine, and holistic medicine, which allowed me to fall in love with the medical profession not as a categorization of body parts, diseases, and pharmacology, but as an opening to the resilient forces of health within.

I stand on the shoulders of great teachers: Jeffrey Bland, MD; Jim Jealous, MD; Elliot Blackman, DO; Ken Lossing, DO; Mark Hyman, MD; Daniel Amen, MD; David Perlmutter, MD; Dale Bredesen, MD; and Paul Harch, MD.

Equally essential are the patients who have seen me at Marin Natural Medicine Clinic and at Advanced Hyperbaric Recovery of Marin, for whom I have shared my knowledge and wisdom and continue to dedicate myself to finding pathways to successful healing. Without them there would be no reason for this book to come into existence. I thank them for entrusting me with their bodies and minds.

Due west about twenty miles of my town are my neighbors, Spirit Rock, an Insight Meditation Center in Woodacre, California, and Esalen, a birthplace for evolving the paradigm for healing. I am eternally grateful, especially to the trees, the soft undulating hills, the Native American land, and the ocean in these places that brought my soul solace.

I'm thankful to Beverly Rubik, PhD, who gave research support for a notion that would not fly in other parts of the world, and to Harry

Jabs, who supported me in measuring photonic coherent light from the body. To my father, whose last words to me were "You come from a family of pioneers, and you are one too." I had always felt safest as a follower; it was not until his death that I nudged myself to the cliff's edge to see what was on a different horizon. He exemplified an unbroken passion in his field of psychiatry.

I thank Vinn Arjuna Martí, founder of Soul Motion, who gave me permission to create through conscious movement. With his guidance I found my inner artist and sense of rhythm in writing. I thank Laura Woodrow, DO, who pored over my manuscript with critical commentary, pushing me to provide more evidence-based research. She is a friend who has woven many threads into my life, from living in the same home as renters at one point, to diving with whales in Tonga, and sharing the intellectual world of medicine. Most of all, when I asked her to do something for me, she gave back a thousand-fold.

I thank my dear soul sister, Barbara Karlsen, for her support on a long road and our many Saturdays writing together. She displayed a love for her work and how it came through the writing process in a way I had never witnessed before or known was possible. I think I learned from her how to write from a wholly authentic and fully integrated place. I thank the patients who never came back because they didn't really understand the reasons for supplements and labs; without them, I wouldn't have written this book. I also thank the ones who did understand and who shared their newfound health and hope.

I give thanks that my keen mind and smart, hardworking brain recovered from all its injuries and that I was curious enough to learn more about the body and healing than I ever was taught in medical school. I feel forever indebted to Janine Thill, the managing director of Advanced Hyperbaric Recovery of Marin, who not only strongly nudged me into the hyperbaric oxygen chamber, catapulting my brain to reach its fullest recovery into sharpness again, but also for her suggestion to "write my own book," which I now have. I thank the osteopathic physicians who helped my brain heal and my community of friends who encouraged me to keep going on my path.

In particular, I thank Anodea Judith, best-selling author, for her encouragement for me to write and teach. She saw in me something I couldn't quite see in myself. To Ernie Hubbard, I bow in gratitude for holding communion with my heart, soul, and mind while I wafted from severe self-doubt and befuddlement over everything from taking on the role of "author" to the details of the graphics and permissions process with a wood crafting tool in hand like a master carpenter. Ernie steered me through the white waters of my sense of urgency and pressure to write this book and get it done in the midst of a full-time medical practice. He has been and continues to be an angel at my back, front, and sides.

I also thank my mother for giving me the gift of life and instilling in me a sense of value around higher education, as well as a German sense of discipline. Her profession as a nurse was a bedrock in her life, as was her meticulous intellect. Her pursuit of higher philosophical and theological study also influenced my knack for swimming in wide waters of thought … the kind that you need to go in when you practice medicine "outside of the box." I thank my grandfather for his marriage to medicine as a noble path of service. He traveled halfway across the world to pursue his medical degree at the Edinburgh University of Medicine in Scotland, far from his homeland of China, and to help during the horrors of WWII from the jungle of British North Borneo. I am grateful for his example of fortitude for all he endured.

Last and not least are the solid workhorses that pull the cart forward, without whom the package would never arrive. Thank you to Nina Shoroplova, leading editor, who pulled me through a much longer path than I thought it would be with eternal patience and steady sure-footed editorial steps. She took me through the fields of "writing" that I had wanted to avoid and encouraged me to do more pruning than forever planting. The wheels of my carriage were Geoff Affleck, who created a program that gave me a guidepost on "how to write a book." Without him my concept would've remained a bunch of Word documents kept inside a cold steel computer drive. He gave a living presence to what I wanted to transport out into the world through words on a written page. Geoff's organized and generous-hearted approach made it all entirely possible.

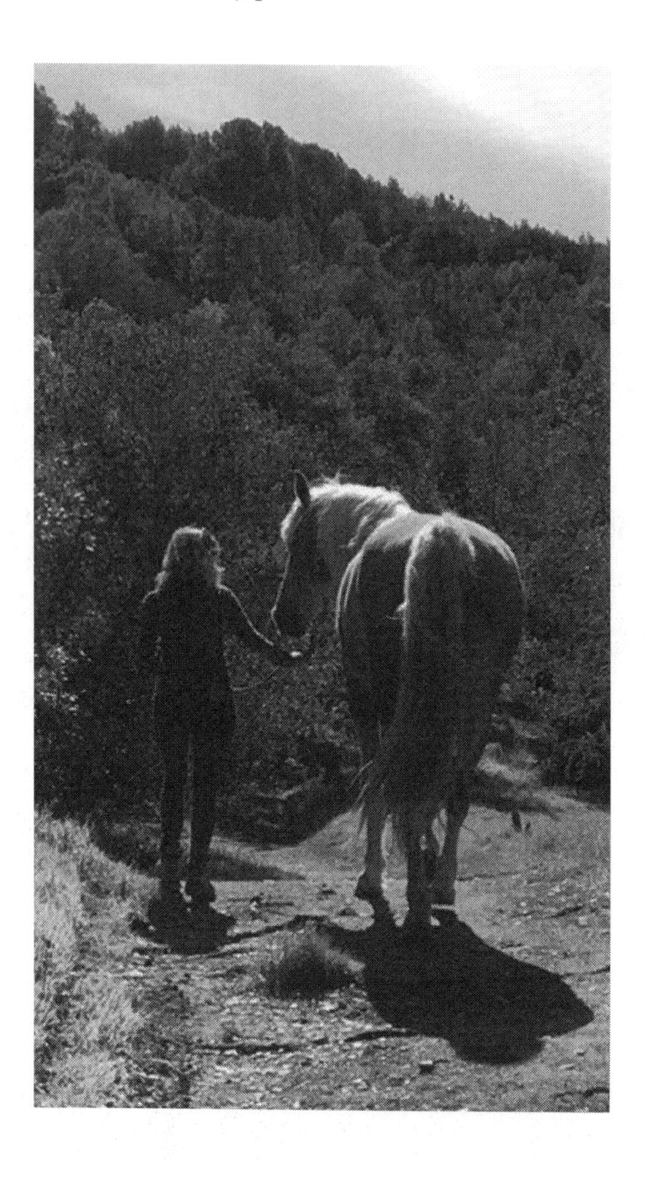

NOTES

1. www.alzheimers.net/resources/alzheimers-statistics/
2. Ibid.
3. www.nami.org/Learn-More/Mental-Health-By-the-Numbers
4. www.aap.org/en-us/about-the-aap/aap-press-room/pages/Childhood-Disability-Rate-Jumps.aspx
5. www.cdc.gov/ncbddd/adhd/data.html
6. www.ncbi.nlm.nih.gov/pmc/articles/PMC2621042/
7. www.ncbi.nlm.nih.gov/pmc/articles/PMC4013121/
8. Wan Y, Zheng J, Wang F, et al. "Fish, long chain omega-3 polyunsaturated fatty acids consumption, and risk of all-cause mortality: a systematic review and dose-response meta-analysis from 23 independent prospective cohort studies." *Asia Pacific Journal of Clinical Nutrition*. 2017;26(5):939-56.
9. Bo Y, Zhang X, Wang Y, et al. "The n-3 polyunsaturated fatty acids supplementation improved cognitive function in the Chinese elderly with mild cognitive impairment: a double-blind randomized controlled trial." *Nutrients*. 2017;9:1.
10. Freeman, MP, Hibbeln, JR, Silver, M, et al. "Omega-3 fatty acids for major depressive disorder associated with the menopause transition: a preliminary open trial." *Menopause*. 2011;18(3):279-84.
11. www.sciencedaily.com/releases/2006/11/061113180236.htm
12. Jurenka, JS. "Anti-inflammatory properties of curcumin, a major constituent of Curcuma longa: a review of preclinical and clinical research."
13. www.ncbi.nlm.nih.gov/pmc/articles/PMC5796761/
14. www.ncbi.nlm.nih.gov/pubmed/20047325

15. www.sciencedaily.com/releases/2015/03/150330112227.htm
16. www.ncbi.nlm.nih.gov/pubmed/15228991
17. foodrevolution.org/blog/food-and-health/best-and-worst-foods-to-prevent-stroke
18. www.ncbi.nlm.nih.gov/pubmed/24335167
19. journals.lww.com/jhypertension/pages/articleviewer.aspx?year=2009&issue=04000&article=00017&type=abstract
20. "Differential responses to NMDA receptor activation in rat hippocampal interneurons and pyramidal cells may underlie enhanced pyramidal cell vulnerability." *European Journal of Neuroscience.* January 2006, 22(12):3077-90. doi: 10.1111/j.1460-9568.2005.04497.x
21. Ibid.
22. Rosanoff A, Weaver CM, and Rude RK. "Suboptimal magnesium status in the United States: Are the health consequences underestimated?" *Nutrition Reviews.* (2012) 70(3):153-164. doi: 10.1111/j.1753-4887.2011.00465.x
23. Afsaneh Rajizadeh, Hassan Mozaffari-Khosravi, Mojtaba Yassini-Ardakani, Ali Dehghani. "Effect of magnesium supplementation on depression status in depressed patients with magnesium deficiency: A randomized, double-blind, placebo-controlled trial." *Nutrition.* 2017 Mar;35:56-60. Epub 2016 Nov 9. PMID: 28241991.
24. www.webmd.com/vitamins/ai/ingredientmono-1003/selenium
25. Xuefeng Liu, Ana Baylin, Phillip D. Levy. "Vitamin D deficiency and insufficiency among US adults: prevalence, predictors and clinical implications." 2018 April;119(8):928-936. PMID: 29644951.
26. Sayeed, I, Turan, N, Stein, DG, Wali, B. "Vitamin D deficiency increases blood-brain barrier dysfunction after ischemic stroke in male rats." *Exp Neurol.* 2019;312:63-71. doi:10.1016/j.expneurol.2018.11.005
27. info.bioticsresearch.com/researchforum/review-the-role-of-vitamin-d-and-lipoprotein-receptor-related-protein-in-amyloid-clearance-and-brain-health
28. www.ncbi.nlm.nih.gov/pmc/articles/PMC5242290/
29. www.ncbi.nlm.nih.gov/pubmed/29107506
30. www.cell.com/cell-metabolism/fulltext/S1550-4131(15)00224-7
31. Hertoghe, Thierry. *The Hormone Solution.* New York: Harmony Books, 2002.
32. n.neurology.org/content/68/12/945.short
33. europepmc.org/article/med/20584515

34. www.cdc.gov/media/releases/2016/p0215-enough-sleep.html

35. www.ted.com/talks/jeff_iliff_one_more_reason_to_get_a_good_night_s_sleep

36. *Endocrinology and Metabolism Clinics of North America.* 2013 Sep;42(3):617–634. doi: 10.1016/j.ecl.2013.05.001

37. www.ncbi.nlm.nih.gov/pubmed/26043918

38. *Ecology Society of America.* 1997. www.biologicaldiversity.org/publications/papers/Medicinal_Plants_042008_lores.pdf

39. Born, Todd A. "Safe, Effective, Natural Solutions to Mood Disorders." *Townsend Letter.* October 2019.

40. Masayuki Hashiguchi, Y Ohta, M Shimizu, J Maruyama, M Mochiz. "Meta-analysis of the efficacy and safety of Ginkgo biloba extract for the treatment of dementia." *Journal of Pharmaceutical Health Care and Sciences.* 2015;1:14. Epub 2015 Apr 10. PMID: 26819725.

41. C Kongkeaw, P Dilokthornsakul, P Thanarangsarit, N Limpeanchob, C Norman Scholfield. "Meta-analysis of randomized controlled trials on cognitive effects of *Bacopa monnieri* extract." *Journal of Ethnopharmacology.* 2014;151(1):528-35. doi: 10.1016/j.jep.2013.11.008

42. Benson, S, et al. "An acute, double-blind, placebo-controlled cross-over study of 320 mg and 640 mg doses of *Bacopa monnieri* (CDRI 08) on multitasking stress reactivity and mood." *Phytotherapy Research.* 2014;28(4):551-9.

43. www.greenmedinfo.com/article/ashwagandha-may-be-effective-enhancing-both-immediate-and-general-memory-peopl

44. www.ncbi.nlm.nih.gov/pmc/articles/PMC4266989/

45. *Microglia.* Khan Academy. www.khanacademy.org/science/health-and-medicine/nervous-system-and-sensory-infor/neural-cells-and-neurotransmitters/v/microglia

46. Maes, M, Kubera, M, and Leunis, JC. "The gut-brain barrier in major depression: Intestinal mucosal dysfunction with an increased translocation of LPS from gram negative enterobacteria (leaky gut) plays a role in the inflammatory pathophysiology of depression. *Neuro Endocrinol Lett.* 2008;29(1):117-124. pubmed.ncbi.nlm.nih.gov/18283240/

47. Majewski, MS, et al. "Pesticides in Mississippi air and rain: a comparison between 1995 and 2007." *Environmental Toxicology and Chemistry.* 2014 Jun;33(6):1283-1293.

48. sustainablepulse.com/2014/02/19/roundup-linked-global-boom-celiac-disease-gluten-intolerance/#.Xh9UjSN6pPY

49. Shaw, William, and Pratt-Hyatt, Matthew. *Townsend Newsletter*. January 2017, no. 402.

50. HN Kim, Y Yun, S Ryu, Y Chang, MJ Kwon, J Cho, H Shin, HL Kim. "Correlation between gut microbiota and personality in adults: A cross-sectional study." March 2018. doi: 10.1016/j.bbi.2017.12.012

51. Dickerson, Faith, Severance, E, Yolken, R. "The microbiome, immunity, and schizophrenia and bipolar disorder." *Brain, Behavior, and Immunity*. May 2017. doi: 10.1016/j.bbi.2016.12.010

52. Messaoudi, M, Lalonde, R, Violle, N, et al. "Assessment of psychotropic-like properties of a probiotic formulation (*Lactobacillus helveticus* R0052 and *Bifidobacterium longum* R0175) in rats and human subjects." *British Journal of Nutrition*. March 2011. doi: 10.1017/S0007114510004319

53. foodrevolution.org/blog/what-does-gluten-free-mean/

54. www.ncbi.nlm.nih.gov/pubmed/28223206

55. "Researchers study links between gut bacteria and brain's memory function." *GeekWire*. February 16, 2018. www.geekwire.com/2018/microbiome-memory. Accessed 15 May 2019.

56. Kharrazian, Datis. *Why Isn't My Brain Working?* p. 188.

57. Ibid. p. 187.

58. *Neuroglial Cells*. YouTube. www.youtube.com/watch?v=hxbaEJWXMW4

59. Reilly, R, McNulty, H, Pentieva, K, et al. "MTHFR 677TT genotype and disease risk: is there a modulating role for B-vitamins?" *Proc Nutr Soc.* 2014 Feb;73(1):47-56. doi: 10.1017/S0029665113003613. PMID: 24131523

    Neggers YH. "Increasing prevalence, changes in diagnostic criteria, and nutritional risk factors for autism spectrum disorders." *ISRN Nutr.* 2014 Feb 13;2014:514026. doi: 10.1155/2014/514026. eCollection 2014. Review. PMID: 24967269

    Nazki FH, Sameer AS, Ganaie BA. "Folate: metabolism, genes, polymorphisms and the associated diseases." *Gene.* 2014 Jan 1;533(1):11-20. doi: 10.1016/j.gene.2013.09.063. Review. PMID: 24091066.

    Schwahn, B, and Rozen, R. "Polymorphisms in the methylenetetrahydrofolate reductase gene: clinical consequences." *Am J Pharmacogenomics.* 2001;1(3):189-201. Review. PMID: 12083967.

Sánchez-Marín, B, and Grasa, JM. [Methylenetetrahydrofolate reductase (MTHFR) C677T polymorphism in ischemic vascular disease]. *Rev Neurol.* 2006 Nov 16-30;43(10):630-6. Review. Spanish. PMID: 17099857

60. Vojdani, Aristo. "Environment and Alzheimer's." *Townsend Letter.* October 2019, p. 32. www.townsendletter.com/article/435-alzheimers-environment-lifestyle-factors/
61. Tracey, Kevin J. "The Inflammatory Reflex." *Nature.* vol. 420, 12/2002, pp. 853-859.
62. Ibid.
63. www.surgeryencyclopedia.com/Ce-Fi/Cerebrospinal-Fluid-CSF-Analysis.html#ixzz5oOt6Z1Mb
64. Fujita K, et al. "Hydrogen in drinking water reduces dopaminergic neuronal loss in the 1-methyl-4-phenyl-1,2,3,6-tetrahydropyridine mouse model of Parkinson's disease." *PLoS One.* 2009 Sep 30;4(9):e7247.
65. Li J, et al. "Hydrogen-rich saline improves memory function in a rat model of amyloid-beta-induced Alzheimer's disease by reduction of oxidative stress." *Brain Research.* 2010:152-61.
66. Mizuno K, et al. "Hydrogen-rich water for improvements of mood, anxiety and autonomic nerve function in daily life." *Medical Gas Research.* 2018 Jan 22;7.
67. www.ewg.org/pfaschemicals/what-are-forever-chemicals.html
68. www.ewg.org/skindeep
69. www.ewg.org/foodscores/content/bpa_bombshell_industry_database
70. iaomt.org/
71. www.ncbi.nlm.nih.gov/pmc/articles/PMC1868496/
72. www.ewg.org/research/bpa-bombshell
73. today.agrilife.org/2018/07/04/texas-am-agrilife-study-shows-bpa-risk-factor-for-inflammatory-bowel-disease/
74. www.sciencedaily.com/releases/2016/09/160920130828.htm
75. www.sciencedaily.com/releases/2013/06/130612173330.htm
76. factor.niehs.nih.gov/2012/5/science-bpa/index.htm
77. www.scientificamerican.com/article/bpa-free-plastic-containers-may-be-just-as-hazardous/
78. ehp.niehs.nih.gov/doi/10.1289/ehp.1003220

79. www.ncbi.nlm.nih.gov/pubmed/23213291
80. www.iaomt.org
81. infraredsauna.com/why-is-sauna-detoxification-important/
82. jwsaunas.com/infrared-sauna-detoxification/
83. www.ncbi.nlm.nih.gov/pubmed/23213291
84. www.ncbi.nlm.nih.gov/pubmed/28633297
85. www.ncbi.nlm.nih.gov/pubmed/27932366
86. *Townsend Letter*, June 2015, p. 50.
87. Dai, DF, et al. "Mitochondria and cardiovascular aging." *Circulation Research.* 2012;110(8):1109-1124.
88. Tampolsky, MA. "The mitochondrial cocktail: rationale for combined nutraceutical therapy in mitochondrial cytopathies." *Advanced Drug Delivery Reviews.* 2008 Oct-Nov;60:13-14:1561-1567.
89. Tsagaris, V, and Liapi-Adamidou, G. "Serum carnitine levels in patients with homozygous beta thalassaemia: a possible new role for carnitine." *The European Journal of Pediatrics.* 2005 Mar;164(3):131-134.
90. journals.lww.com/acsm-healthfitness/Fulltext/2013/05000/HIGH_INTENSITY_CIRCUIT_TRAINING_USING_BODY_WEIGHT_.5.aspx
91. "The Scientific 7-Minute Workout." *The New York Times Magazine.* May 12, 2013.
92. *The Scientific 7 Minute Workout Video.* YouTube. www.youtube.com/watch?v=Jru5B044HOs
93. jamanetwork.com/journals/jamaneurology/fullarticle/799078
94. Harch, Paul. "Oxygen and Pressure Epigenetics: Understanding Hyperbaric Oxygen Therapy After 355 Years as the Oldest Gene Therapy Known to Man." *Townsend Letter.* April 2018, p. 33. www.townsendletter.com/article/oxygen-and-pressure-epigenetics-understanding-hyperbaric-oxygen-therapy-after-355-years-as-the-oldest-gene-therapy-known-to-man/
95. Moss, M, Scholey, A, and Wesnes, K. "Oxygen administration selectively enhances cognitive performance in healthy young adults: A placebo-controlled double-blind crossover study." *Psychopharmacology* 138, 27–33 (1998). Download citation, Issue Date, July 1998. doi: 10.1007/s002130050641
96. link.springer.com/article/10.1007/s002130050641
97. Harch, PG, and Fogarty, EF. "Hyperbaric oxygen therapy for Alzheimer's dementia with positron emission tomography imaging: a case report." *Medical Gas Research.* 2019 Jan 9;8(4):181-184. doi: 10.4103/2045-9912.248271

98. www.nature.com/articles/ncomms11934

99. Rossignol, DA, et al. "Hyperbaric treatment for children with autism: a multicenter, randomized, double-blind, controlled trial." *BMC Pediatrics*. 2009;9:21.

100. Collet, JP, et al. "HBO-CP Research Group. Hyperbaric oxygen for children with cerebral palsy: a randomized multicenter trial." *Lancet*. 2001;357:582-86.

101. Fisher, BH, M Marks, T Reich. "Hyperbaric oxygen treatment of multiple sclerosis: a randomized placebo-controlled double-blind study." *The New England Journal of Medicine*. 1983;308:181-6.

102. Rockswold, SB, et al. "A prospective, randomized Phase II clinical trial to evaluate the effect of combined hyperbaric and normobaric hyperoxia on cerebral metabolism, intracranial pressure, oxygen toxicity, and clinical outcome in severe traumatic brain injury." *Journal of Neurosurgery*. 2013;118(6):1317-28.

103. Wang, SP, et al. "Hyperbaric oxygen combined with donepezil in the treatment of vascular dementia. *Chinese Journal of Physical Medicine and Rehabilitation*. 2009;31(7):478-80.

104. Harch, Paul. "Oxygen and Pressure Epigenetics: Understanding Hyperbaric Oxygen Therapy After 355 Years as the Oldest Gene Therapy Known to Man." *Townsend Letter*. April 2018, p. 33.

105. hyperbaricoxygentherapy.com/testimonials/post-concussion-following-car-accident | hyperbaricoxygentherapy.com/testimonials/rapid-recovery-from-concussion-and-trauma | www.youtube.com/watch?v=zOt_TMSLmDQ&t=35s

106. "BDNF Responses in Healthy Older Persons to 35 Minutes of Physical Exercise, Cognitive Training, and Mindfulness: Associations with Working Memory Function," www.ncbi.nlm.nih.gov/pmc/articles/PMC6135088/

107. Meletis, Chris, and Wilkes, Kimberly. "Mitochondria: overlooking these small organelles can have huge clinical consequences in treating virtually every disease." *Townsend Letter.* June 2015, p. 54.

108. Caufirex, A, et al. "Progesterone prevents sleep disturbances and modulates GH, TSH, and melatonin secretion in postmenopausal women." *The Journal of Clinical Endocrinology and Metabolism*. 2011 Apr, 96(4):E614-23.

109. www.ncbi.nlm.nih.gov/pmc/articles/PMC3004979/

110. www.ajpmonline.org/article/S0749-3797%2898%2900017-8/fulltext

111. *Psychological Bulletin.* 1990, vol. 108, no. 3, 363-382.

112. forestsangha.org/teachings/books/clarity-and-calm?language=English

113. Ramanath M, Bhavananni AB, Trakroo M. "Effect of a 12-week yoga therapy program on mental health status in elderly women inmates of a hospice." *International Journal of Yoga*. 2017 Jan-Apr;10(1):24-28. doi: 10.4103/0973-6131.186156

114. journals.plos.org/plosone/article?id=10.1371/journal.pone.0030253

115. Pall, Martin. *5G: Great risk for EU, US and International Health! Compelling Evidence for Eight Distinct Types of Great Harm Caused by Electromagnetic Field (EMF) Exposures and the Mechanism that Causes Them.* 2018. www.ncbi.nlm.nih.gov/pubmed/29655646

116. Pompei, Pierluigi. "BEMER Electromagnetic Field Therapy in patients with senile dementia: Case reports." 8th International Conference on Natural and Alternative Medicine, September 25-27, 2017, Dubai, UAE. *Scientific Tracks* abstract: *Alternative & Integrative Medicine.* doi: 10.4172/2327-5162-C1-032

117. Importance of Healthy Blood Flow (11-minute video). life.bemergroup.com/8MinuteStory/?utm_source=ALL_PARTNERS_NA_2019_51&utm_campaign=a19a732ab6-

118. www.researchgate.net/publication/338020507_We_Are_What_We_Think_Downregulating_the_Chronic_Stress_Response_with_Technology-Assisted_Mindfulness_Meditation/fulltext/5dfaca5a92851c8364882f8e/We-Are-What-We-Think-Downregulating-the-Chronic-Stress-Response-with-Technology-Assisted-Mindfulness-Meditation.pdf

119. Bostock S, Crosswell AD, Prather AA, Steptoe A. Mindfulness on-the-go: Effects of a mindfulness meditation app on work stress and well-being. *The Journal of Occupational Health Psychology*. 2019;24:127-38

120. www.researchgate.net/publication/232084164_The_Therapeutic_Value_of_the_Human-Animal_Connection

121. www.youtube.com/watch?v=stuZaKB9j7I